NEWLY REVISED EDITION
MORE THAN 170,000 SOLD

D0104832

Heartmates®

A Guide for the Spouse and Family of the Heart Patient

Rhoda F. Levin

> "...a complete and compassionate treatment of the needs and fears of the family of a heart patient. **Heartily recommended**"
>
> **-Harold S. Kushner,** author of *When Bad Things Happen to Good People*

SLIDELL MEMORIAL HOSPITAL
1001 GAUSE BOULEVARD
SLIDELL, LA. 70458

PRAISE FOR

HEARTMATES®

A Guide for the Spouse and Family of the Heart Patient

PRAISE FROM DOCTORS

"Compassionate, intelligent advice for the spouse of a cardiac patient...."

– Dean Ornish, M.D., author of
Eat More, Weigh Less

"... this useful book...is a guide to living as a tourist in the harsh, overpowering world of the hospital. It will be as close a companion as any tour book. It is a guide to the perplexing inner emotional experience of living through a cardiac event with a spouse. Finally, it is a guide to the intimate handling of that most delicate of heart patients, the marriage.

"*HEARTMATES*® brings help on many levels simultaneously. First and foremost, it is a handbook offering guidance for help in dealing with the hospital and medical staff, with feelings, the family, and marital intimacy. It offers suggestions for coping with life-style changes, and it lists resource centers where information is available. There are many brief case examples from the experiences of other cardiac spouses. Finally, interwoven with wonderful delicacy, is the story of the author's experience .... They appear in my memory of the book as trail markers on forest trees."

– David V. Keith, M.D.
Director of Family Therapy, and
Associate Professor in Psychiatry,
State University of New York
Syracuse, New York

BLUDER MORTIST HOSPITAL
BLVE' BLEVARD
BL   TAS

"This book supplies a much-needed lifeline that the cardiac spouse can use as a guide and for reassurance."
– Robert S. Eliot, M.D., F.A.C.C., author of
Stress and the Heart and Is It Worth Dying For?

"A book that has been eloquently written by a woman who has 'been there' and, in addition, I found it a practical approach to many other crises in life, not just heart disease....I realized what a wonderful guide this could be to all those affected by our leading cause of death and disability."
– Allen M. Lansing, M.D., Ph.D.
Director, Humana Heart Institute International

ACCLAIM FROM CARDIAC SPOUSES

"Written professionally and poignantly, HEARTMATES® deals with human fears and confusion — an exceptional coping-guide. It literally was a life-line thrown to me at a most troubling time."
– Muriel Whitaker
heartmate of family therapist,
Carl A. Whitaker, M.D., co-author
of The Family Crucible

"Being a cardiac daughter, a cardiac sister and a cardiac spouse by the age of 27, I highly recommend this book. It will assist your most basic needs while numbed by the trauma of cardiac disease. HEARTMATES® will become a best friend."
– Jeanne Moutoussamy-Ashe
heartmate and widow of Arthur Ashe

"I was parched and your book watered me."
— **heartmate** from Springfield, South Carolina

"...[your] wonderful book...has helped me feel like a human being again rather than a robot."
— **heartmate** from Biloxi, Mississippi

"We farm 800 acres and farrow to finish 1200 hogs a year....I could relate to every word in your book....[it] has been a great help to me."
— **heartmate** from Morristown, Minnesota

"I am writing to tell you that you have probably saved my life....My husband had a major heart attack five years ago....I realized that I have not recovered. Finally, someone understood and I was not going crazy!! You have no idea the relief that brought. I cried and cried and it was the first real cry in five years and it was for ME, finally. I am allowed to have a life. I am allowed to be angry. But most important, I AM NORMAL!

What a change [the book] has made in my life. It has probably saved our marriage of 31 years, too, but that's another...."
— **heartmate** from Kitimat, British Columbia

"Thank you for helping me understand that I am going through a crisis, but that I'm not alone."
— heartmate from Gilbert, Arizona

"It seemed as if by some guiding light your book reached out to me....Since then it has comforted me and kept me grounded."
— **heartmate** from Waynesboro, Pennsylvania

"I feel as though I have my own private support system every time I read segments from your book."
— **heartmate** from North Adams, Massachusetts

"I had thought I was the only one going through these feelings and I couldn't understand what was going on with my body and myself....I must tell you I was not enthused about reading HEARTMATES®; I was not sure if I wanted to hear the truths about heart disease...It's a must to be read by spouses everywhere."
— **heartmate** from Stockton, California

FROM REVIEWS OF THE BOOK

"An important, timely book...."
— **American Library Association Booklist**

"An excellent book...."
— **Library Journal**

"...remarkable account of love, strength and survival will comfort all those who live with the chronically ill."
— **Modern Maturity, magazine of AARP**

"HEARTMATES® is a complete and compassionate treatment of a subject that has been waiting for someone to deal with it: the needs and fears of the family of a heart patient. Heartily recommended."
— **Rabbi Harold S. Kushner,** author of
When Bad Things Happen to Good People

"HEARTMATES® added to my deep appreciation of how my wife supported me at the time of my bypass surgery, and how she continues to support me today. It is a book I recommend highly to heart patients, spouses and medical professionals."

– Joseph C. Piscatella, author of
Controlling Your Fat Tooth and
Don't Eat Your Heart Out Cookbook

"...first a comfort for strange and frightening times, and then a guide through unfamiliar and stormy waters: at the hospital; at home and coping with change....A comprehensive heart guide for heart partners."

– Audrey DeLaMartre
Minneapolis StarTribune

"Interspersing helpful information on such topics as anxiety, communication, family issues, an sexuality with descriptions of her own experience, Ms. Levin offers a combination of factual and helpful information and personal sharing which holds the reader's interest from cover to cover."

– Paul V. Johnson
Caregivers Quarterly

"HEARTMATES® who read this book will identify with it, and healthcare professionals...will obtain greater insights into their patients and their families....This book should be available to heartmates®."

– Judith Schiffert, RN, EdD
Reviewed in the Journal of Cardiopulmonary Rehabilitation

"A much needed, realistic presentation of the complexities of living with heart disease....will be a source of comfort and strength to...cardiac spouses who feel isolated, scared, and alone."

– Rona D. Weinstein
National Cardiac Patients' Support Network

The cases and examples cited in this book are based on actual situations and real people. Names and identifying details have been changed to protect privacy. In some instances case illustrations are composite creations, based on the author's professional clinical experience.

For information about other Heartmates® resources, professional training or motivational speaking, contact Rhoda F. Levin, MSW, at:

Heartmates Inc.
P.O. Box 16202
Minneapolis, Minnesota 55416
(612) 929-3331
Fax: (612) 929-6395

To communicate with us and with other heartmates, e-mail us at:

heartmates@aol.com

or, look for us on the WorldWideWeb, where our url is:

http://www.heartmates.com/

Heartmates®
A Guide for the Spouse and Family of the Heart Patient

by Rhoda F. Levin, M.S.W.

FOREWORD BY

David V. Keith, M.D.
Director of Family Therapy
State University of New York, Syracuse

Heartmates® A Survival Guide for the Cardiac Spouse
© 1987, Rhoda F. Levin
Revised Edition: Heartmates® A Guide for the Spouse
and Family of the Heart Patient
© 1994, Rhoda F. Levin

The trademark, Heartmates®, consisting of the word and the logo, is regis-
tered in the U.S. Patent and Trademark Office, and in other countries, to
Heartmates Inc., Minneapolis, Minnesota, U.S.A.

All rights reserved. Inquiries about the use of the material in this book should
be addressed to: Permissions, MinervaPress, a division of the J.D. Scram Company, P.O. Box 16202, Minneapolis, MN 55416.

Library of Congress Cataloging-in—Publication Data

Levin, Rhoda F.
       Heartmates® A Guide for the Spouse and Family of the Heart Patient
       REVISED EDITION

       Bibliography: p.
       Includes index.
       1. Heart – Infarction – Patients – Family Relationships
       2. Wives   I. Title
       RC685.16L43   362.1'961237   87-11392
ISBN 0-9637795-1-6

Printing History
(First Printing, Prentice Hall Press, Division of Simon & Schuster, October 1987,
ISBN 0-13-385162-1)
(First Pocket Books Printing, March 1989. ISBN 0-671-67899-X)
(Revised Edition, First Pocket Books Printing, October 1994, ISBN 0-671-51095-9)

Cover and interior design: Cottage Communications
Cover art: "New Reality" © 1994 Bonnie S. Barland

This edition is printed on an acid-free paper that meets the American National
Standards Institute Z39.48 Standard.

Manufactured in the U.S.A.

25 20 15 10 9 8 7 6 5 4

*To wounded families
everywhere
and especially to my own children,
Sidney and Deborah, and to their children*

ACKNOWLEDGMENTS

There are many people, here unnamed, who have contributed to my growth and in some way have made this book possible. I am grateful to all of them: those I have worked with as colleagues and clients, those I have known personally, and those who have taught me through their writing. I thank each and all of them. I am especially grateful to:

The many cardiac spouses who trusted me with their stories, their pain, their indomitable strength, and their recovery

Psychosynthesis, its principles and practitioners - it was within that framework that I discovered my sense of purpose

The mentors I've been privileged to learn from - to Harry Sloan for introducing me to psychosynthesis, and to Rene Schwartz, who held me in her wisdom and love, as I searched for my truth

Elisabeth Kübler-Ross, for her courage to cut a professional path that I could walk on and expand from

Ellen Sue Stern, who helped me transform my vision into a physical and accessible reality

Gareth Esersky, my editor at Prentice Hall Press, for believing in the book and giving to it her gifts of clarity and precision

Denise Silvestro, my editor at Pocket Books, for encouraging me to address the special needs of the male cardiac spouse and for her vision in navigating this revised edition

Arlen R. Holter, MD and his staff, for helping me access male cardiac spouses to interview for the new chapter

My friends, who have supported me as a cardiac spouse and as a woman: Bonnie Barland, Pamela Borgmann, Shirley Kaplan, Vonnie Kilkelly, Nancy Lundborg, Chelle Stillman, Harriet Swartz, Sandy Swirnoff, and my sister Judy Mack; and my friends Arnold Kaplan, Marvin Stillman, and Stephen Swartz, for their steadfastness, and their respect for my work

My daughter, Deborah Levin Stillman, who typed and proofed the manuscript, assisted in the preparation and writing of the new chapter in this edition, and continues to give her creative energy to Heartmates® projects. . . for her love.

CONTENTS

PREFACE TO THE 1994 EDITION

It has been seven years since the publication of *Heartmates® A Survival Guide for the Cardiac Spouse*. Heart disease continues unabated, and is our largest disabler and killer. Recent technological advances and pharmaceutical miracles have increased survival rates substantially. Although heartmates® has yet to become a household word, there may now be more than twenty million of us.

What's new in heart disease? What's new is that women are afflicted with heart disease too. The number of balloon angioplasties done in our country has risen from a few thousand in 1979 to more than 300,000 in 1991, the most recent year for which there are statistics, according to the American Heart Association. Of that number of angioplasty procedures, 100,000 recipients were women. Although women generally develop heart disease some ten years later than men, by age fifty-five heart disease is the number one killer of women. About half of the 500,000 people who die every year of heart attacks are women. In contrast approximately 45,000 women die from breast cancer, the disease women fear most.

What's new about heartmates? In this revised edition of *Heartmates®* special attention is paid to male heartmates who are growing in numbers close to the number of women heart patients. The printing of this revised edition also gives me the opportunity to look back over these years to appreciate and recount progress, and to clarify what still needs to be accomplished for cardiac spouses and families.

Healthcare professionals at every level have embraced concepts outlined in the Heartmates® resources, coming to understand that when someone is given a cardiac diagnosis, goes through a procedure, or has a heart attack, the event involves more than the heart patient. The patient is a part of a larger unit, the family system, and the lives of all family members are changed forever by a cardiac event. As healthcare professionals expand their definition of who the patient is, they are beginning to treat the whole cardiac family.

A new field of study, dealing with the vicarious victims of trauma, legitimizes the issues and needs of cardiac families experiencing a shocking and unexpected cardiac event.

Cardiac rehabilitation today generally includes Heartmates® principles and practices as a normal component of established programs. Many cardiac professionals report great satisfaction assisting cardiac spouses with their unique and universal needs. Nurses, social workers, and chaplains have welcomed the resource of the book, utilizing it as the foundation of cardiac spouse educational programs in hospitals and clinics all across North America. *Heartmates®* is now available in French and German, and we are working on requests for Spanish and Hebrew editions.

I have been privileged to travel throughout the United States, Canada, and Israel training cardiac professionals and addressing cardiac couples. I have heard remarkable stories from cardiac families about the challenges they have encountered and triumphed over. Many newspaper and journal articles, as well as radio and television interviews, have clarified and provided franchise for some of the issues cardiac families face.

Of the thousands of cardiac couples I have addressed, never once, except in Reno, Nevada, in March of 1993, has a patient or spouse asked a question about sex in relation to cardiac recovery. So I know that our work is not done; issues about communication and renewed physical intimacy are a fundamental concern to people, but still difficult to express openly.

Understanding that family support and emotional factors play a significant role in the heart patient's as well as the cardiac family's recovery, Marion Laboratories commissioned me to create a series of educational videotapes for cardiac spouses and families to view in the hospital. These video programs, given by them to 5,000 hospitals as a public service in 1989-1990, have provided widespread recognition of the serious crisis sustained by cardiac families, and have been utilized to aid the heartmate's recovery.

Canada, with full support by Nordic Laboratories (a subsidiary of Marion Merrell Dow Inc.), has adopted the Heartmates® resources for its cardiac families. Every clinic and hospital across the country has the video programs in French or in English. Nordic Laboratories has also given hospitals the two hundred page professional manual, The Cardiac Family Recovery Program Training Manual for Administrators and Facilitators, so that hospitals could provide appropriate programs and classes for their cardiac families. Early in 1994, the Heartmates® resources were endorsed by the Canadian Cardiovascular Society and the Canadian Association of Cardiac Rehabilitation.

Without Nordic and Marion Laboratories' support, literally hundreds of thousands of cardiac families would still be isolated and unprepared. Instead, because of their commitment, families are learning to accept heart disease as a part of their reality. Able to emerge from the shock, they can begin to live life anew, with new skills and understanding.

Some of the most gratifying of my personal experiences has been that many, many heartmates® have written to me, appreciating the book or the video programs and expressing that they feel more understood and less alone. They have let me know specifically what has been of practical help and what has given their spirits a needed boost. Their words have helped to enrich this new and revised edition. The letters help me to remain focused; they remind me of the importance of continuing to work to bring the heartmate vision to fruition, to persevere so that heartmates everywhere will be recognized and supported as we go about the tasks of healing our wounds, adjusting to our new family reality, and rebuilding our heartmate relationship.

I hope this book will help you with the experience of being a heartmate in recovery. Celebrate each milestone and give yourself permission both to grieve your losses and to find joy in each precious day.

Rhoda Levi

Rhoda F. Levin
Minneapolis
October, 1994

FOREWORD

Fantasies and nightmares produce more unresolved fear than reality. Reality, faced in isolation, can be a nightmare. The reality of a heart attack is unclear because of the way it distorts and fragments the living patterns of a family. Even when the medical staff members suggest that it is a mild heart attack, the family must deal with the distress of unanswered and unanswerable questions. What is the likelihood of death? What will be the extent of disability? Fragments of information from diverse sources cause confusion and despair.

Ms. Levin's useful book, written for those with a spouse who has experienced a cardiac event, will be of great consolation to many. It is a guide to living as a tourist in the harsh, overpowering world of the hospital. It will be as close a companion as any tour book. It is a guide for providing home care for patients recovering from cardiac disease. It is a guide to the perplexing inner emotional experience of living through a heart attack with a spouse. Finally, it is a guide to the intimate handling of that most delicate of heart patients, the marriage.

Heartmates® brings help on many levels simultaneously. First and foremost, it is a handbook offering guidance for help in dealing with the hospital and medical staff, with feelings, the family, and marital intimacy. It offers suggestions for diet, coping with life-style changes, and it lists resource centers where information is available. There are many brief case examples from the experiences of other cardiac spouses. Finally, interwoven with wonderful delicacy, is the story of the author's experience with her husband's two heart attacks and successful bypass surgery. These personal samples are used to illustrate what is too ambiguous to describe. They appear in my memory of the book as trail markers on forest trees.

While the bright light of technological advance in medicine illuminates disease processes, improves survival rates, and reduces the disabling components of serious illness such as coronary artery disease, the human despair at the center of the experience remains hidden in darkness. The families of heart patients are subject to massive, long-term, often unacknowledged distress. The process leaves the family brittle and lacking resilience.

Case example: Several years ago the Swenson family was referred to me because Bill, age thirteen, the second of five children, had been arrested for vandalizing cars in their upper-middle-class neighborhood. It was not until the third family therapy interview that we discovered that the father, age forty-eight, had had a coronary one year previously. It was no accident we were not told, because the family was under the father's strict orders not to speak of his heart attack. In his words, it had been a "mild" heart attack and "could have no possible effect" on the family. Over his protestations, his wife and children described their concern about their husband and father. They were angry that he remained seriously overweight and continued his heavy smoking. The mother said she had not had a full night's sleep since his heart attack, and every time he became upset with the children's fighting, she was fearful it would precipitate another attack. The father was very upset with me for encouraging his family to talk about their experiences. "It has nothing to do with my son's problems," he repeated emphatically. Yet the family's relief at being able to talk openly was obvious. The tough, taciturn thirteen-year-old vandal told freely about his fears that his father might die. Mr. Swenson refused to bring his family back for another interview. Six months later, the family doctor who had referred them told me that Bill had become a starter on the hockey team, and was back on the honor roll.

This case review gives an example of some less obvious side effects of coronary artery disease. *Heartmates®* would have been invaluable to Mrs. Swenson in providing a support for her reality, which was at odds with her husband's. Her reality included her own anxiety symptoms, the distress she could see in their children, and her fantasies about what would happen if he died. His reality included only his doctor's suggestion that it was a mild heart attack and that he could resume his normal work schedule. He had no idea what his wife and children were experiencing and his denial of death was ludicrous.

Coronary artery disease can be a catastrophic and/or chronic illness, causing problems for the whole family. Health, both physical and psychological, is a function of a family's morale, the family's heart. The clinical tools for helping families under stress have evolved in the mental health professions, but have not been integrated into the medical world. Books like this one will educate the families of patients so that they can be more aware of the implications that serious illness in a family member has for them. As families come to understand the way they are affected by illness, it may lead to changes in the way medical practitioners view the experience of illness. If illness is placed in the context of family living patterns rather than in the simpler individual context, then families can be treated so that patterns of family living do not have a detrimental effect on a member who is ill. Instead, the patterns of family living can be guided so as to enhance recovery for both the patient and the family.

David V. Keith, M.D.
Director of Family Therapy and
Associate Professor in Psychiatry,
State University of New York
Health Science Center
Syracuse, New York

Introduction

As the spouse of someone who has survived the sudden onset of heart disease, you are in a special category, one relatively new in our society. In the last twenty years, advanced medical technology and pharmaceutical discoveries have revolutionized the treatment of heart disease. Hardly a day goes by that we don't hear of a new study clarifying risk factors or announcing another technological breakthrough. Five hundred bypass surgeries and as many angioplasty procedures are done in our country every day. Billions of dollars are spent on medical treatment and research. The predicted number of heart attacks annually in the United States is 1.5 million. Of these, more than one million will survive. Each year the number of cardiac spouses grows. Today there may be as many as twenty million of us.

Strange as it seems, it may be easier in some ways to be widowed than to be the spouse of a recovering heart patient. There are role models for a widow's behavior, and appropriate ways to express difficult emotions. People respect the time it takes for the widowed to adjust to the changes in their lives.

Cardiac spouses have no role models, teachers, or mentors. No one, professional or friend, can tell you what specific changes you will face as a cardiac spouse, and yet change is your reality.

When my husband had his first heart attack, I felt totally unprepared. I was forty-three, an urban mother, wife of an architect, and well established in my second professional career.

Marsh and I were typical 1950s high-school sweethearts. He was the football hero and I the adoring coed. The future looked unlimited from where we stood. We were both bright and talented. College provided us with an additional layer of confidence, optimism, and idealism. I felt like Wonder Woman: healthy, invincible, and protected by her magic bracelets. It never dawned on me that I was marrying anyone less than Superman.

Our first adventure in the early 1960s was to leave the safety of Minneapolis and make our way in the Big Apple. Marsh, a Coast Guard officer, was stationed at the Battery in New York City. I taught English in an all-black junior high school in a well-to-do New Jersey suburb. We involved ourselves in the desegregation movement: Marsh through sports and I through my work with adolescents. It was exciting and satisfying to conclude those years believing that our lives were meaningful. We were committed to living life as an adventure and making the world a better place. I believed that if we just worked hard and believed in justice we could do anything. I had felt neither danger nor limitation.

In 1966, Marsh's dad died of a heart attack. Three months later, we left for Tunis, Tunisia, to serve in the Peace Corps. We were of the generation that could respond to John F. Kennedy's call to serve: a little too old to be flower children and still too young for his assassination to suggest danger or mortality for ourselves. Getting by the dangers, real or imagined, of being Jewish in an Arab country during the Six-Day War, and of being pregnant and having our first baby two continents away from home and family, added to my sense of invincibility. We were strong and resilient, and we returned to Minneapolis in 1968 unscathed and triumphant.

During our early thirties, our adventures were focused within our individual professional fields. Marsh's energy went toward his work in architecture. I went back to school to earn a graduate degree in social work. We had a second child, and struggled somewhat separately and silently with the problems of keeping careers and family intact. My mother died when I was thirty-five, and that experience taught me that I was vulnerable. If my mother could die, then I could too. But death and illness still seemed very far away. I never considered at that time that Marsh could die.

Approaching our forties, having achieved success in our careers, our restlessness and our search for meaning were renewed. Marsh tried a career change; my idealism uprooted us again, and with our two little ones, we left Minneapolis for San Francisco to work in the human potential movement.

By the fall of 1980, I was ready to return home. We hadn't changed the world; we had seen more violence and danger than ever before. We were disappointed and disillusioned. Wounded by the reality, but still believing in our own resilience and invincibility, we started over again.

Our expectations of what we could and should accomplish were scaled down; we were maturing. We were concerned about rebuilding a safe and secure home back in Minneapolis for our young family. Marsh returned to architecture; we bought a house and I began to rebuild my therapy practice. On the night of November 16, 1981, as we lay in bed watching "Monday Night Football," Marsh turned to me and said, "Don't get scared, but I think I'm having a heart attack." That moment was the last of my old life, a life in which I had thought we would live and triumph over everything and every situation, forever. It was also the first moment of my new life, a life that included being a cardiac spouse.

Marsh was having a heart attack that night. Nine weeks later he had a second heart attack. Fortunately both left him with minimal heart damage. Regaining his strength, Marsh returned to work full time and to a life with few physical restrictions. He went faithfully to a cardiac rehabilitation class three times a week, which also functioned as his emotional support group.

I recovered from the shock of becoming a cardiac spouse at age forty-three, but I was more confused than ever before in my life. Every aspect of my life was in flux: All my old beliefs had failed me, my security was lost, even my daily life-style was different. Marsh wasn't invincible and neither was I. My feeling of being in control of the life and well-being of our family had vanished. My experience as a clinical social worker helped me identify that I was in crisis. But wherever I turned, I felt alone. I couldn't find a support group to attend. There wasn't one book available that spoke to the issues I was facing.

I stumbled around, trying to deal with the uncertainty and the real changes, and after a year and a half decided to start a program that could help me and other cardiac spouses. Ironically, I was scheduled to present my program to a local hospital's cardiac rehabilitation team that very week in the late fall of 1983 when Marsh's heart health radically changed. He was scheduled for an angiogram on Wednesday, I presented the Heartmates® program on Thursday, and Marsh had quadruple bypass surgery on Friday. Recovery for each of us and for our relationship took longer psychologically than physically. It was disappointing and very difficult to have to start over again.

I have written this book because I believe recovery is possible, for me and for you. In this book I share what I've learned from my own experience and from the opportunity to work with many cardiac spouses in the Heartmates® program. My hope is that you will identify with and be strengthened by reading about others who struggle with issues similar to your own.

My intention has been to write for all cardiac spouses, men and women alike. At the present time, less than one third of all cardiac spouses are male, but their numbers continue to rise. In relation to my use of language, I have chosen to subordinate semantics and the limitations of our language to my message. After considering the use of he/she, I chose to use the traditional "he," trusting that neither "he" nor "she" will be alienated or offended.

There has been up to now a lack of recognition about the emotional dimension of the cardiac crisis and heart disease. It is my hope that cardiologists, thoracic surgeons, primary care and family physicians, as well as cardiac nurses and cardiac rehabilitation professionals will read *Heartmates®* and will continue the progress already begun: to close the gap between physical medicine and caring for the whole person, including the family system. I wish for all of us that competent and compassionate care becomes the standard for patients, their spouses, and families.

Full recovery depends on a balance between the healing of the physical being and the psyche. For that reason, this book combines and interweaves practical information, psychological support, and emotional guidance.

Each cardiac spouse is unique, and every cardiac situation is different. This book does not propose a specific cure for living with the realities of heart disease. It does include suggestions, tips, and tools. What works for one person or couple may not be effective for others. Consider all specific suggestions as ideas with which to experiment, suggestions to be molded to fit your own personal needs and situation.

The book is arranged chronologically, beginning in the hospital and moving through aspects of recovery. But because of the ongoing nature of heart disease, the setbacks and plateaus that complicate recovery, you may want to reread the early chapters often, even if you are a longtime veteran.

At another level, the book goes from the elementary to the complex, from the simple and more obvious changes, to deeper issues and questions. Themes in later chapters are recovery and the healing of relationships with your mate, your family, and yourself. These issues are fundamental to the ultimate quality of our lives, but for most of us, they are the last to be recognized and dealt with.

The challenge of the cardiac crisis is facing the reality of your situation, letting go of what is lost, and developing new ways to live that enhance the quality of your life. My experience has deepened my belief that relationships are what matter most. I have strengthened my commitment to myself and to my marriage. I try to appreciate each day as it comes and cherish the precious gifts of life and love.

I hope that you will rely on this book as you journey through your cardiac crisis. Heartmates® is meant to be such a guide. It is also a reminder that you are not alone. Accept my support and the shared experience of the many others in this book who reach out to stand with you as well, as you deal with the difficulties and opportunities of being a heartmate.

At The Hospital

My heart racing, I park and run through the darkness toward the double doors marked Emergency. Where is my husband? The ambulance he arrived in stands empty and there is no sign of him. Only an hour ago we were safely curled up in bed, watching TV and comparing notes on the details of our day. His sudden chest pain and an urgent call to 911 have led me to this door, where I stop, take a deep breath, and realize I don't know what to do.

Once inside, I am jolted by the glare of artificial light, medicinal smells, and an operator's strident voice repeatedly paging doctors. I need to get my bearings, gather my composure, and figure out a plan. But I'm frantic, not knowing whether Marsh has had a heart attack or is even alive.

I approach the registration desk and I am directed to Admitting. A woman behind a computer says to be seated, she will call me. The minutes tick by. I try to keep from screaming at her to hurry up. Doesn't she know this is an emergency? Finally she begins the ritual list of questions establishing identity, financial responsibility, and the nature of the complaint. I search my mind for Marsh's social security number and my wallet for insurance infor-

7

mation. I can't believe I'm wasting time doing this when I should be with Marsh. When she's finished, I'm motioned back to the waiting room to resume my vigil.

After an hour, I am told that Marsh is being taken to Coronary Care. I ride with him on the elevator, but when we reach the fifth floor I'm waved away to wait in the family lounge. I'm not sure what's happening. It seems certain that Marsh has had a heart attack, but how sick is he? When can I see him? Where is the doctor? Should I stay all night or go home to be with our children and try to get some sleep? How can I possibly sleep? If I leave, will he die?

My body is numb. My mind races a million miles an hour with questions coming so fast and furiously that one begins where the last one leaves off. I'm tempted to escape this nightmare but I don't know how. Instead, I brace myself and walk into the coronary unit. Rules are posted at the nurses' station. Visitors are allowed ten minutes each hour, only one person at a time. My eyes are riveted by a half dozen monitors, each silently recording ongoing lines that are images of the patients' heartbeats. On one, the green line is zigzagging uncontrollably in an ominous pattern. What if it's Marsh's? What should I do? I tell myself to take it easy; I don't even know how the machine works.

The nurse calmly informs me that Marsh is resting comfortably and that I can see him for just a few minutes. Everything is quiet and controlled here, the sounds absorbed by carpeting. I imitate the nurse's measured tone, lowering my voice before entering Marsh's room.

Now, after two excruciating hours, I stand at Marsh's bedside. I don't know what to say. Marsh is all wired up. There's an oxygen tube in his nose and an intravenous line dripping liquid into his wrist. He is attached to a machine that gives a digital readout of his pulse; it is equipped with a miniature version of the screen at the nurse's desk. Again I stare at the critical green line that mysteriously makes its way from left to right, reappearing again and again.

Marsh says he knows he has had a heart attack, but that he isn't in any pain. He asks me to take care of

some arrangements at the office and jokes about cancel-
ing his breakfast date since he obviously won't be there.
His ashen skin and frightened eyes belie his businesslike
manner and his humor. I'm not sure how to act and
whether or not to show how worried I am. Before I've had
a chance to sort out my feelings, the nurse signals that my
time is up. I lean over to kiss Marsh, careful not to disturb
the lifesaving equipment.

On my way out, I stop at the desk for reassurance
that Marsh will be okay if I leave. The nurse says it's fine
to call any time, day or night. I find my car in the lot and
drive home, where I collapse onto our bed and sleep fit-
fully until dawn.

Whether your introduction to being a cardiac
spouse started with your mate's heart attack or bypass
surgery, *your* crisis began as all do, suddenly and without
warning. While heart disease develops over a long period of time, a cardiac crisis happens in an instant. You
might have noticed gradual signs, such as your spouse's
shortness of breath, or pallor that is unlike his familiar
ruddy complexion. But nothing prepared you for the terrifying split-second when you witnessed his heart attack.
Nor for the seemingly routine checkup that indicated the
immediate need for an angiogram, angioplasty, or bypass
surgery. At that moment, you were catapulted into a new
and frightening reality. With no time to absorb what had
happened and no way to know what was ahead, you were
propelled into action and forced to deal with a life-and-
death crisis.

In many ways, a cardiac crisis is similar to other
life-threatening emergencies. However, cardiac spouses
share the unique experience of being in a crisis precipitated by someone else's illness. Your mate is in crisis too,
but the experience is not the same. You suddenly find
yourself in a situation entirely beyond your control that

threatens your security and will change your future. Unless you have medical training, you are faced with a foreign vocabulary of medical terms you can barely pronounce, let alone understand.[1] You may have to decipher this technical information in order to make decisions with far-reaching consequences on behalf of your mate. And to top it all off, the one person on whom you rely is totally unavailable. Instead of operating as part of a team, you must deal with this all on your own.

In a crisis, the initial reaction is often numbness. Cardiac spouses describe a sense of being removed from reality, as if they are walking around in a dense fog. One spouse described her astonishment at the difference betweeen her experience in the hospital and the larger world: "I found myself in a very specialized environment...where quiet efficiency was the order of the day. When I emerged from the hospital at the end of the day, I was surprised to see that the world was still there - buses were running, people were laughing and talking, and life was going on as usual." During the first few days, you may have trouble concentrating, making decisions, and carrying on conversations with relatives and friends. These are typical reactions. The body shuts down in response to shock to prevent being overwhelmed. It serves as a protective shield, masking the intensity of feelings, allowing you to continue functioning. This is usually a temporary reaction that quickly passes. At this time it's wise to preserve your energy, and handle only those tasks and decisions that absolutely cannot wait.

Living in Limbo

Once the numbness wears off, you will probably become fearful. The most compelling fear is that your spouse won't survive. Despite medical evidence to the contrary, it is natural to associate a heart attack with death. And even though bypass surgery has an impressive track record, it inevitably evokes fear and anxiety. Anxiety, often as not, manifests itself physically. During the first days, while you wait for conclusive information about your mate's condition, you may feel like a tightly wound spring, ready to snap at the slightest provocation. Other symptoms include loss of appetite, trembling, shallow breathing, or insomnia. One spouse noticed his arm ached and realized he had been constantly clenching his fist. Another developed a nervous habit of biting her lip. Fear paralyzes some people, makes others withdrawn, and causes still others to become overactive, aimlessly pacing the corridors of the hospital or chattering incessantly.

The hours spent waiting during surgery can be the most difficult of all. While it may help to have close friends and family around for distraction and support, ultimately you are alone with your fears. Thoughts about the outcome of surgery bring up a set of survival questions that keep you holding your breath. Will he be in that small percentage that doesn't make it through bypass surgery? Will his heart beat on its own after being connected to the heart-lung machine? Will he breathe when they remove the respirator? Will he get pneumonia? How long will the new arteries work, or will they just collapse? There's no way to speed up time, and the surgeon's words, "The surgery was successful; all vital signs are stable," are only a partial remedy.

Seeing Marsh lying in the intensive care unit was dramatically different from anything I could have imagined. There were neither windows nor clocks in the cu-

bicle and time felt indefinitely suspended. Marsh's hold on life seemed very tenuous. Every part of him was hooked up to something. He was at the center of a whirlwind of activity. Skilled, efficient nurses moved swiftly in and out, executing complex life-sustaining procedures. I knew that morphine protected Marsh from pain, but he was restless and straining against the respirator. His hand and arm, still chilled from surgery, felt like a stranger's. All the while the regular rhythm of the monitors reassured me with its beep . . . beep . . . beep. I returned to the waiting room totally shaken by what I had seen. Marsh couldn't even breathe on his own. How would he ever be healthy and whole again?

Once the initial crisis passes, your worries continue, intensified by the unknown nature of heart disease. While you are relieved that your mate has survived, new questions arise. What are the details of his condition, and what is the long-term prognosis? Will your spouse have constant pain? Will he be dependent on medication? Is he going to be an invalid? Will he be able to work, to travel, to lead an active and fulfilling life? What are the chances of another heart attack?

Most of us have a hard time coping with the unknown. *Learning to live with uncertainty is one of the greatest challenges for the partner of someone with heart disease.* Knowing that your mate is in competent professional hands can alleviate fear. While it's essential to get all the information and medical guidance you need, it's also important to recognize that even the most gifted physicians cannot foretell the future. The best they can provide are percentages for recovery. Medicine, for all its awesome accomplishments, is still a limited science.

Your anxiety will diminish as you become more secure about your mate's survival and as the repercussions of his illness become clear. In the meantime, voice your concerns. In some hospitals, trained social workers and chaplains are available to help you through this traumatic time. Acknowledging your fear to someone or to yourself can reduce its power, as shown in the following story.

Ruth, a soft-spoken woman in her early fifties, drove her husband forty miles to the hospital emergency room. After his examination, she was told to follow him and his entourage of medical staff to the intensive care unit. At the big double doors she was stopped and told to wait outside. No one explained what was happening. Ruth sat alone in the silent corridor for close to an hour. During that time she considered every possibility. She didn't think she would ever see Ralph alive again. She reviewed the highlights of their thirty years together, thinking about what he meant to her and how much she would miss him. She recalled their dreams and tried to imagine pursuing them alone. She even planned his funeral, picturing herself there with their three sons.

The doors of the intensive care unit swung open and a nurse emerged. Ruth, lost in her own thoughts, was startled. The nurse told her that Ralph was doing well and all vital signs were stable. She burst into tears of joy and relief. But the hour Ruth had spent waiting was a turning point in her life. She had prepared herself emotionally for the loss of her husband and confronted squarely the idea of living as a widow. Ruth rose to go to her husband feeling strengthened and confident in her ability to cope with whatever would be their new reality.

In the midst of crisis, fears intensify and get blown out of proportion. The urgency of the situation makes it almost impossible to keep things in perspective. Lack of information increases dread and permits you to imagine worst-case scenarios. We are so accustomed to having physicians provide clear answers that any vagueness or gray area can be interpreted as bad news. Some people naturally cope with the unknown by adopting a positive attitude—they know survival is a given. Others are more likely to envision the worst. When told that ninety-eight percent of the people who have bypass surgery survive, they automatically place themselves with the remaining two percent.

Anxiety in the face of the unknown is a normal and appropriate response, as long as it doesn't impair your ability to function. Go ahead exercising a cautious optimism: the combination of a positive outlook with a realistic appreciation for the gravity of the situation. That way you can hope for the best and still be prepared to cope with any contingencies.

Making Yourself at Home

As you struggle with your fear about your mate's survival and recovery, you need to deal simultaneously with a new and strange environment. Trading the familiarity of home for the alien atmosphere of the hospital further distorts your reality and gives you the feeling of disorientation. Your schedule is completely out of kilter, and your sense of time is governed by hospital routine: rotating shifts, the return of the latest test results, and the doctor's rounds. For all intents and purposes, you have taken up residence at the hospital. You may spend periods of time at work or at home, but your mind and your heart are somewhere else.

How do you handle the hospital? First, you must recognize what part the hospital plays in your emotional experience. On the one hand, it's a relief to see your spouse safely ensconced, attended by professionals who can prolong, and, in some instances, save his life. On the other hand, the hospital system is not designed with your needs in mind. The physical layout, regimented pace, and antiseptic environment is geared toward maximum care and increased productivity. Its primary purpose is to accommodate the patients and medical staff.

It goes without saying that your first priority is your mate's recovery. *However, you too have needs, basic human needs that arise in a crisis, including: the need to belong, the need to be needed, the need for information, and the need for support.* In order to feel comfortable, you must first understand the lay of the land. Find your way around, know the location of the lounge, the telephone, the gift shop, the coffee shop, and the chapel. Doing so will contribute to a semblance of order. It's frustrating to find yourself on the Employee Only elevator en route to the supply room, missing a long-awaited ten-minute visit with your mate. And the fact that most family lounges are hidden away in an obscure corner adds nothing to your feelings of connection and belonging.

Once you get your bearings, the next step is to understand the inner workings of the system. This is what I call "cracking the code." A hospital is a unique world, with its own language, customs, and culture. Your aim is to effectively maneuver and negotiate on behalf of yourself and your spouse. This necessitates learning the procedures, vocabulary, and chain of command.

At times you may feel frustrated or in the way. Everyone else rushes around doing an important job, while you hurry up and wait: for visiting hours, for a few minutes with the doctor, for test results, for rehabilitation meetings. In some ways your needs seem at cross-purposes with the running of the hospital. You trust your cardiologist's competence more when you see how busy he is. But because of his pressing schedule, he makes his rounds before you can get there in the morning or in the only half hour you leave to get a cup of coffee. And when you finally catch up with him, you have forgotten the one question you meant to ask. You admire the nurses' ability to handle so many things at once. But the fact that they're so busy makes you hesitant to bother them with your questions. After a while, it all starts to seem like a conspiracy to keep you in the dark.

There is nothing you can do to change the nursing staff's style, but *you have every right to ask them questions.* If there never seems to be an appropriate time to do so, set up a specific time to discuss your concerns. It's unlikely that you are going to change your doctor's schedule. But you might try calling his office to find out when he will be on hospital premises or make a formal appointment instead of anxiously waiting for his appearance.

Cardiac spouses often perceive the hospital staff as a lifeline, but this can make you feel very dependent on them. Such dependence can, in turn, cause you to be especially careful in your relationships with the nurses and doctors. You worry about asking too many questions or being labeled pushy or demanding. You might be hesitant to arrange for the privacy you know will make your mate more comfortable. You may be afraid of making a wrong move, inadvertently doing something to antagonize the nurses and jeopardize your spouse's care.

Whether or not it's justified, it doesn't take long to get the idea that if you're "good," and wait patiently without making waves, your mate will benefit from first-class service by the staff. One cardiac spouse never came to the hospital without bringing candy for the nurses. Another always prefaced her questions with an apology, fearing the nurses would think she was stupid or wasting their time. Another felt hesitant to tell the nurses that her mate was someone of great age and dignity, and that it would be more respectful to call him "Mister" than to use his first name.

Many cardiac spouses are reluctant to express their opinions, thinking that their input will be construed as interference or doubt.

Early in Marsh's hospitalization, I wrestled with the conflict between my desire to be seen as a "cooperative spouse" and my need to participate in his care. In an educational session with the coronary care nurse, Marsh and I were shown a chart of "mets," the units of energy expended in each physical activity. It covered the period from the heart attack through six weeks of recovery, listing the graduated activities that would ultimately lead to resuming a normal life.

The following day, Marsh was moved to a cardiac recovery unit. A nurse appeared and informed him that he had bathroom privileges. I knew she was wrong. According to the mets chart, bathroom privileges were several days off. Although it wasn't ten yards away, I reacted as if Marsh were being encouraged to sprint around a track or take an extra base on an infield single. As much as I wanted him back on his feet, part of me wished he could permanently remain in coronary care and never again do anything that took any mets at all. Why tempt fate? Better he should do nothing more active than breathe, love me, and live.

I didn't want the stigma of "trouble," but I was determined that Marsh not get out of bed until the chart permitted. I found the charge nurse, waited until she was free, and told her that Marsh did not have bathroom privileges and wouldn't for several days. Once I said this, my fear subsided. In its place a new dread appeared: if this mistake could be made, I'd better stay watchful and alert in case a bigger or more dangerous one occurred. If it were necessary, I'd move in and stand guard twenty-four hours a day.

Combating Helplessness

It's natural to feel helpless when you are caught up in events beyond your control. In some ways you truly are helpless. Nothing you can do will turn back the clock. You can neither change nor ignore the fact that your spouse has heart disease. There's no way to reverse the risk factors and life-style choices that contributed to this crisis. And unless you are medically trained you are incapable of providing the technical care that's required. It's important to acknowledge these realities, but it's equally valuable to recognize your power.

Most of us endow physicians with too much power. In a crisis we're apt to expect physicians to work miracles. Terrified, we expect them to have all the answers and never make mistakes. Once we make the doctors omnipotent, it's difficult to have appropriate expectations of them. And by giving up so much power to your doctor, you diminish your own. If you have a question or idea, you may stifle it, thinking, "I've never been to medical school," or, "If the doctor thought it was necessary, he'd have recommended it." What you don't take into account is that *no physician knows everything*. Regardless of how smart or dedicated a doctor is, no one can keep up with every new development in a field. Your doctor is the medical expert, but you know more about your mate than anyone else does. And no one cares as much as you and your husband about his full recovery. Sharing your knowledge can be crucial in planning his recovery program with the staff.

You can increase your power and self-respect by educating yourself about heart disease. The more you know, the more you will be able to contribute to your spouse's recovery. Christina, an avid reader, came across a ten-year study of a medication thought to reduce cholesterol rates. A year earlier, her husband, Paul, had undergone bypass surgery and she wondered if the newly available medication might be a significant addition to his exercise and diet program of recovery. Christina clipped the article and showed it to their doctor, who followed up and prescribed the medication.

Sometimes we withhold valuable information because we feel intimidated or shy. But your intimate relationship with your spouse makes it especially important for you to speak up. Stuart, a quiet and intuitive man, felt terribly uneasy sitting beside his dozing wife, Kim, the first night following her bypass surgery. Despite assurances that Kim was in stable condition, he was seized with an irrational sense of foreboding. Something was wrong, and while he couldn't put his finger on it, the feeling was impossible to dismiss. When a nurse passed, Stuart asked her to check Kim, who indeed was developing post-surgical complications. Within minutes, emergency measures were taken and a potential disaster prevented.

Information is another factor in counteracting helplessness. It is your need,[2] your right, and your responsibility to have access to all the available data.

Under state law, we are protected by a "Patients' Bill of Rights." (Ask for a copy of your bill of rights from your nurse or hospital social worker.) Among twenty-six sections of the Minnesota bill are four that are especially pertinent to cardiac family members:

1. Patients have the right to be treated by the staff with courtesy and respect for their individuality.
2. Patients have the right to be given complete and current information concerning their diagnoses, treat ment alternatives, risks, and prognoses, in language

they can be expected to understand.
3. Patients (including a family member) have the right to participate in the planning of their health care.
4. Patients have the right to a prompt and reasonable response to their questions and requests.

HEARTMATES® HOSPITAL QUESTIONS

The following list is a guide for asking questions and gathering information. As you read over the items, note the questions that concern you the most, and add new ones as you go along.

Heart Attack

1. What is a heart attack?
2. What does heart damage mean?
3. How long does recovery take?
4. Will my spouse need open heart surgery?
5. What causes a heart attack?

Medications

1. What is the medication supposed to do?
2. What are the potential side effects?
3. How long will the drug need to be taken?
4. How frequently is it taken?
5. What happens if a dose is missed?
6. What is the generic name of the drug?
7. What are the reasons for changes in medications?
8. What should we do if he can't remember having taken his pills?

Surgery and Procedures

1. What is angioplasty? What is bypass surgery?
2. When is a procedure or surgery indicated?
3. What are the advantages? The risks?
4. Who is best qualified to do the surgery?
5. Where can we get a second opinion?
6. How soon should the procedure or surgery be done?
7. How long does it take to recover from angioplasty? From bypass surgery?

Recovery

1. When will my mate be able to come home?
2. What life-style changes should be made?
3. Will he have to change his job or retire early?
4. What kind of emotional reactions should I expect from my spouse? How long will he be depressed or angry?
5. Will we be able to resume sexual activity? When? Are there any dangers involved in having intercourse?
6. How often should we schedule appointments with the doctor? Will the hospital provide any ongoing support? Whom should I call to answer my questions?

Your list of questions is undoubtedly lengthy and will change daily. Put them in writing to help remember them, and to mark the significance of your concerns and bolster your confidence. Once you have compiled a list, decide who can best respond. Some questions should be directed to your family doctor or your cardiologist. Others require the expertise of the nursing staff, the exercise physiologist, the nutritionist, or a veteran cardiac spouse.

You are absolutely entitled to all the information you need. If the answers you receive are too vague, such as, "Oh, that's nothing to worry about" (easy for you to say), or, "Time will take care of that" (how much time?), be prepared to ask again. In some instances, an unsatisfactory answer may be precipitated by an unclear question. You may need to be more specific. In some cases differences in family, religious, or ethnic background between you and the professional staff may make communication more difficult or complex.

Some doctors are comfortable answering questions and are sensitive to your feelings and concerns. Others are defensive, unresponsive, and noncommittal. They may brush off your questions for a number of reasons, including time pressures, lack of communication skills, and discomfort discussing issues that are painful or ambiguous.

Ideally, your doctor is someone whose medical knowledge you trust and with whom you are personally comfortable. More likely, as in any relationship, there are compromises. Your doctor may be a respected expert in cardiology, but he may have limited experience in a variety of surgical procedures. He may enjoy the best medical reputation in town, while his bedside manner may leave something to be desired.

What matters is knowing what will make you feel most secure. Out of loyalty to your doctor, you may feel that you should unconditionally accept his judgments. In truth, your only obligation is to pursue a course of treatment that will facilitate your mate's recovery, provide for your peace of mind, and honor the human dignity of you both. If you're unsure after his diagnosis, seek a second opinion. If the two conflict, get a third. If you and your mate are ill at ease with your doctor, look for another.

Bridging Communication

Assertive action enables you to be useful in another way. When someone you love is hurting, it's normal to want to help. During the hospital stay your contribution seems superfluous; from the moment your mate arrives, professionals and technology take over and you are relegated to the background. You would do anything in the world to help, but it feels as if there's nothing to do.

Actually, there are many ways to be of use. There are at least two ways in which you can act as a bridge immediately following surgery: by acting as an intermediary between your mate and the busy professional staff, and as a connection to reality for your mate.

Right after surgery your spouse is totally vulnerable. The presence of a respirator and throat tubes make even verbal communication impossible. He has no way to make his simplest needs known. One practical suggestion is to use a "magic slate" (the children's toy) to help your mate express what he wants. There are things you can do for him yourself. Moistening dry lips, moving a sheet that's pulling on a tube, or readjusting a pillow can be important for both of you. Other things may require the expertise of the nurse. Your spouse may be anxious about a machine that has changed the rhythm of its "beep," and you can ask the nurse to explain.

Checking on medications is another way to act as a bridge. You can actively participate in your mate's care by becoming familiar with the name, dosage, and purposes of drugs being administered. Your spouse will feel some control over his own care if he can monitor his medications for dosage accuracy and take them on time. Both of you will feel more secure if you understand how the medications work.

The first days following surgery are distinguished by a drug-induced haze that protects your spouse from pain, but may also cause him alternately to doze, be easily startled, be out of touch with reality, or say bizarre things. One woman reported that her husband thought he was being experimented on in a concentration camp. Another man admonished his family to hurry to the midnight buffet on the promenade deck of their cruise ship.

Your presence is significant to your mate because it is a symbol of stability and reality at a time of extreme confusion and vulnerability. With no other frame of reference available to him, you are your husband's connection to his earthly roots, his home, his family, his recovery, his life. Add powerful medication to an absence in the cardiac care unit of windows or clocks, and the already strange environment can be overwhelming. Simply telling the patient the time and whether it is day or night can provide him with an important reality check. Letting him know how long he's been there may furnish significant direction for his return to the world of life and the living.

Nourishing Yourself

Being a bridge is both a gift to your mate and a way to reduce your helplessness. By giving, you increase your power. But it's equally important to be able to receive. In a cardiac crisis, everyone's focus is understandably on the patient. However, you, too, are physically and emotionally vulnerable. Your daily schedule has been disrupted, you are spending most of your waking hours at the hospital, you are deeply affected by your mate's illness, and you are trying to juggle your spouse's needs with the other demands in your life.

Adequate rest and proper nutrition are two things that are often neglected in a crisis. This can lower your resistance and make you more susceptible to illness. You must eat regularly and get sufficient sleep. Hospital food is usually marginal, so it's a good idea to eat a nutritious breakfast at home. You might also pack a bag lunch and bring healthy snacks to eat in the family lounge. You need to keep your energy and spirits up, and, besides, a shared snack can be an ice-breaker in an otherwise tense situation.

Even if you are normally sedentary, take a walk at least once a day. Take a break from the confines of the hospital and get some fresh air. Just being in the outside world can replenish your resources.

I can't emphasize enough the importance of support. With the amount of pressure you are under, you run the risk of becoming depleted or resentful unless you nourish yourself too. This is an appropriate time to let yourself be taken care of by friends and relatives who are willing to bring food, accompany you on a walk, or visit with your spouse so that you can take a break. If ever you need and deserve support, it's now. There's no reason to try to do it all alone.

Before You Leave...

Many hospitals offer cardiac patients and spouses an educational program to provide information about diet, exercise, risk factors, stress, and sexuality. These classes are usually held while your mate is still hospitalized, with the purpose of preparing you to go home.

In order to facilitate this process, let your nurses and doctors know what you need. It's safe to assume that the hospital staff members want to help, that their goal is to promote healing. That doesn't make them mind readers. Tell the staff if you have forgotten a detail from an earlier meeting and would appreciate hearing it again. If you are having trouble concentrating, say so. Be specific about areas that concern you, and keep on asking questions until you get the answers. If you feel embarrassed by your lack of knowledge, remember that you are in a totally new situation. These sessions are for *you*, so be sure to take advantage of the information and support.

Later, let the staff know how practical and worthwhile the educational sessions were. Your feedback is bound to benefit cardiac families in the future. And the staff, committed to quality care, will appreciate your perspective.

A good educational and support program will:

• Keep educational meetings short (no more than ten to fifteen minutes).
• Provide time for each couple to discuss the information with each other during or after each session.
• Make a question box available for individuals who are uncomfortable speaking in a group.
• Offer at least one meeting for cardiac spouses to identify their most pressing questions and concerns regarding preparations to take their spouses home.
• Provide clear and simple handouts covering the material discussed.

As you two move into the recovery phase, you may want to participate in an educational program that meets regularly. This can be very valuable as you make the transition from the acute crisis into the next stage, which brings its own new issues and concerns.

The hospital experience is only the beginning of a long-term situation heralded by the cardiac crisis. Issues that begin here will follow you home. You will have to learn to deal effectively with the medical community; it's just one part of life with someone who has a chronic condition. A positive way to approach this is to develop an ongoing relationship with your hospital staff members.

Since heart disease is incurable, this may not be your only time at the hospital. Nine weeks after Marsh's first heart attack, he had a second one. Two years later, sudden changes in his condition brought him back to the hospital for an angiogram followed by bypass surgery. Should you need to return to the hospital, you'll feel more at home if you have participated in educational programs and meetings in the interim.

In time, you will adjust more and more to living with uncertainty, but there will continue to be areas over which you have no control. You do not have the power to eradicate your spouse's heart disease or eliminate its effects on your life. Your primary goal, as you anticipate bringing your mate home from the hospital, is to be prepared to support his recovery and yours.

● ● ● ● ●

CHAPTER NOTES

1. Refer to Appendix A for diagrams of healthy, damaged, and bypassed hearts. See Glossary for clarification of medical terminology.
2. It's validating to hear other healthcare professionals state what I know both from the experience of being a cardiac spouse, and from working as a clinical social worker. At a 1994 seminar on Family Health and Chronic Illness given by William J. Doherty, Ph.D., master

teacher and ground-breaking clinician, he stressed that when there is a diagnosis or an acute event, families usually rally around, and they need access to "what's going on"; they need information.

On The Road To Recovery

*T**he phone hasn't stopped ringing all morning. Every one wants to know when Marsh will be home so they can come over to see him. Soon everything will be back to normal, and our lives will be just the same as they were before his heart attack. Driving to the hospital, I feel eager and excited. The days have seemed like forever. I'm grateful that there were no complications, that this nightmare is almost over.*

I arrive in Marsh's room at the same time as his favorite nurse. Upbeat and professional, she carries a thick packet of papers which she ceremoniously turns over to me. In it are exercise diagrams and schedules, cholesterol tables, and scores of heart-healthy recipes. The nurse gives us a last reminder about avoiding undue stress, and checks to make sure that Marsh has his medications for this afternoon. Finally, she hands me several prescriptions and instructs me to have them filled immediately.

I feel somewhat reassured by her orderliness and efficiency, but I'm a little nervous about taking Marsh home. I'm not sure if he's strong enough to wait in the car while I stop at the drugstore, or if I should drop him off at home and then go to fill the prescriptions. I don't know what to do, and my head is full of conflicting details and directions. I'm beginning to feel as though I've accepted a "Mission Impossible" assignment without fully realizing how difficult and dangerous it might be.

The nurse insists on pushing Marsh in a wheelchair. She assures me that he's fine, that it's hospital policy, but I feel as if I'm taking home an invalid.

The back seat of the car is filled with gifts, books, and six large plants that Marsh accumulated during his stay. We're finally on our way home, the two of us, surrounded by symbols of life and love from all his well-wishers.

We stop at our neighborhood drugstore, and I rush in to get the pills. It seems to take forever to count out a few pills and label the bottles. The total comes to almost forty dollars. I'm shocked at the cost, but I quickly write a check and rush back to Marsh. He looks a little worn. I think about "undue stress" as I drive toward home and decide not to mention how expensive the prescriptions are.

Tears of joy fill my eyes as the kids throw their arms around Marsh to welcome him home. They stick around to keep us company while I unpack. I arrange the plants all around the bedroom because I want the "healing green" to be near Marsh. But it still looks like a sick room, with the hospital water pitcher, the medicine bottles, and the pile of new books.

By this time Marsh says he is tired and is going to take a nap. It's hard for me to imagine how he could be tired from just riding home from the hospital, but I say nothing and leave him to sleep.

I sit down with my packet of recipes and instructions, but I can't concentrate. I'm drained, but too wound up to relax. I feel disappointed that we haven't really talked or celebrated his homecoming. For days we have lived in public view, and I have had to share him with doctors, nurses, and technicians. The logical voice in my head begins to instruct me about what I should be thinking and feeling. "Calm down," it says. "You should lighten up, feel grateful, say a prayer of thanksgiving. Everything will be just as it used to be."

It wasn't. That first day home was only the begin-
ning of the emotional upheaval that followed. Little did I
know how much Marsh's heart attack had already
changed my life.

What happened to me and what is happening to
you is this: You have lived through the beginning phase
of a crisis. You are beginning to adjust to changes that
began abruptly and are beyond your control. These
changes have already affected you, and will continue to
have an impact on your life in ways that you cannot yet
predict. Even homecoming, the anxiously awaited reunion
with the family, turns out to be far different from the anticipated "return to normal." Although you don't have
heart disease, every part of you is vulnerable to the cardiac crisis.

The myth is that everything will be the same as it
was. The truth is that *nothing will ever be the same again.*

New Ingredients

Any life crisis brings change on many levels. Early
in the cardiac crisis the basic elements of your life-style
are the most noticeably affected. At a time when you especially need nourishment and rest, you are coping with
new dietary requirements and disrupted sleep. No aspect
of your life is immune to this crisis. Your work schedule,
leisure time, and social life have been interrupted and
altered. Your primary relationship, too, is in transition.
And your personal goals and dreams, beliefs and values,
are undergoing change as a result of your mate's heart
disease.

Adopting a heart-healthy diet is the number one
concern for most couples in the early stage of recovery.
Before you became a cardiac spouse, you were probably

only vaguely aware of diets that may have prevented heart disease. You may have gradually shifted your family away from red meats and toward fish and fibers. A heart-healthy diet is not much different from the general trend toward nutritious eating. But for the cardiac spouse it involves more than wanting to be fashionable or fit. It feels as if it is a matter of life and death. And that puts a lot of pressure on you.

Before Marsh's heart attack, our diet was primarily Midwestern: meat and potatoes. I salted liberally, and never checked frozen foods for sodium, fat, and cholesterol content. Meals, which were previously a casual affair slipped in between our teenagers' various extracurricular activities, became a major undertaking.

I had to learn to cook all over again. I found myself unhappily spending hours in the kitchen absorbed in recipes, meal planning, and food preparation. It reminded me of being a newlywed, trying to impress my husband with delicious and healthy meals. I experimented with herbs and spices to replace the deadly salt I had been warned against. I searched for recipes that would transform broiled pike into barbecued ribs.

There is general agreement that diet may improve recovery and prolong a heart patient's life, but a new food plan requires time and planning. It can't happen overnight. One extra milligram of salt in your spouse's soup will *not* cause him to keel over on the spot. You may feel guilty about the eating habits you have taught your family, or you may even believe that your cooking method was a primary cause for your spouse's heart disease. But only in recent years has a correlation between diet and heart disease been seriously considered. Years ago, "low-sodium" was hardly a household word. So there's no reason to blame yourself now. To cry over whole, not skim, milk, is neither productive nor constructive.

Use your new knowledge positively now and in the future. But don't throw away all the food in your freezer when your mate gets home from the hospital. During a time of crisis, when everything is upset and upsetting, you need to take things slowly and make changes gradually. As much as you can, let the past go, and focus on what you can do now.

Preparing healthy meals is a way to contribute to your mate's recovery. For many couples, making dietary changes together can be a statement of shared commitment and an opportunity for closeness. While a cardiac diet may seem to lack variety or spice, it offers a potential second chance at life.

A new food plan is a positive signpost on the road to recovery, but it may unfortunately also become a dangerous detour. For some couples, changing eating habits is a source of conflict and stress. It's common for partners to disagree about strict adherence to a food plan and how significant a factor of heart disease it is, when it comes down to selecting what foods to eat.

This is one area where being a cardiac spouse is especially difficult. You want to do everything in your power to help your mate stay on a healthy diet, but your spouse is also an adult, who is responsible enough to choose what he eats wisely.

Adjusting to a rigid new diet requires effort and discipline. Most recovering heart patients take a break from the approved list of foods now and then. Certainly you will worry about your mate's commitment to a healthy diet. But everyone deserves an occasional treat.

Overly critical comments or controlling behavior may reflect your fear of losing your spouse. Arguing about food can also be a way for both of you to blow off some steam and express some of the stress of your situation.

Suzanne took a three-month leave of absence from her job as a computer programmer in order to care for her husband, Jim, who was recovering from surgery. She devoted herself to cooking delicious, healthy meals and helping Jim stick to his diet. If they were going out to eat, Suzanne either called ahead to check the menu or brought along a separate meal for Jim. One night Jim arrived home with half a dozen chocolate brownies that he proceeded to devour. Suzanne, bristling with anger, burst out with, "Chocolate. You may as well eat poison."

Suzanne's perfect recovery plan was ruined. She didn't want Jim to be deprived of pleasure, especially since it was the first time he had broken the diet since the surgery. But watching him eat six brownies made her realize how terrified she was of losing him.

Monitoring your mate's diet can be a way of trying to maintain control in a situation that is overwhelming and actually beyond your control. In a time of crisis, when the usual ways of expressing love and caring are interrupted, the preparation of food takes on more significance. In most relationships, sharing food connects people emotionally. Women have been brought up to communicate their feelings and show their love by preparing and serving meals.

Many cardiac spouses say they sense a lack of appreciation for their efforts. Angelina, the cardiac spouse of a proud Italian restaurant proprietor, spent night after night making heart-healthy meals. After years of pasta in cream sauce, she assumed that Carl found the cardiac fare boring and bland. One day Angelina drove clear across town to a gourmet grocery where she bought special herbs for dinner. All through the meal she waited for Carl to comment on her Chicken Rosemary. He ate silently. Finally, she asked. His response: "I prefer it plain."

Angelina was crushed. She interpreted Carl's reaction as a personal rejection of her and her cooking. In fact, his lack of enthusiasm probably had little to do with Angelina or her efforts to please him. More likely it was a statement about his own change in values regarding food, an indication of depression, or of his effort to cope with his new diet. (And many a recovering heart patient becomes apathetic about food, or decides that it is less of a priority in life.)

During this transition, communication is every bit as important as cuisine. There is no diet plan that will assure immortality, no one way to prepare food or eat it that is right for a particular couple. But you and your mate can talk about the dietary changes that heart disease has brought to your household and negotiate how to cope with this ongoing adjustment in your lives.

FOOD ISSUES TO DISCUSS WITH YOUR HEARTMATE

Questions to ask are:

- How important an issue is diet to you?
- How do you feel about sticking to the diet?
- Who is responsible for changing and controlling the diet?
- How do you want to handle exceptions ("cheating") to the diet?
- What can you do if the two of you disagree?
- Are you willing to eat a heart-healthy diet?
- How can you share responsibility for a new food plan?
- How can you best take care of yourself in relation to food and diet?
- What support do you want and need to help you with this diet reform?

It may be new for you to think so seriously about how and what you eat and feed your family, but understanding your beliefs and feelings about food will prove useful. You have the opportunity to follow a healthier food plan, one that is more satisfying and nourishing to both of you. Because diet is a risk factor, the emotional stress attached to it is high. But we all have to eat, and the cardiac spouse can choose a brand new, healthy approach to food.[1]

Getting Your Rest

In order to provide your mate with support, it is essential for you to maintain your own health and well-being. In caring for the patient, you may unconsciously place your own needs for sleep and healthy eating second. Cardiac spouses often report that they are too worried or anxious to sleep. Interrupted or fitful sleep is a natural reaction to stress. Once the initial numbness and shock wear off, it is normal to remain on guard and tense. If your whole life can change in an instant, it might happen again at any time. Your entire being responds to the continuing threat of danger. The initial crisis has passed, yet it is difficult to relax and, sometimes, to sleep.

There probably isn't a cardiac spouse anywhere who hasn't awakened abruptly in the middle of the night, ready to dial 911. I spent many nights holding my breath, listening for the sound of breathing, waiting anxiously to see the blanket move gently up and down. It triggered my memory of being a new mother, always listening with one ear for the baby.

Recovering cardiac patients often sleep fitfully and need naps during the day. This change may be temporary, caused by the new medications and the trauma of going through a heart attack or cardiac procedure. Irregular sleep or changes in your mate's sleeping patterns aren't necessarily danger signals or something to be concerned about. Still, it may take some time before you will be able to fall asleep peacefully, confident that your partner is all right.

You may also be worried that lack of sleep will be a setback to recovery. Having been told that rest is an essential part of the healing process may increase your anxiety about your partner's restlessness. *But worry doesn't help.* Although it took many months, I finally stopped asking my morning worry question, "How did you sleep last night?" For me, Marsh's report of how many times he had awakened in the night, or of how long he lay tossing and turning, counting and recounting the meager number of hours slept, only served to aggravate my concern. We'd both been awake, and we'd worried together, but it did nothing to improve his sleep or mine.

Eventually, the patient's new sleep patterns will become more routine and less frightening to you. In the meantime, you need to get all of the rest you can in order to restore your emotional and physical energy. This may mean cutting back on some of your activities or taking the phone off the hook so that you can grab a nap. A short period of conscious relaxation (see appendix B for an exercise designed to help you relax) can soften tense muscles and calm nervous feelings. Deep breathing works wonders when you feel too tense to sleep. Take in a long, deep breath through your nose, and exhale slowly and completely through your mouth until you feel that all the air is out of your lungs. Repeat this five to eight times. Try using these relaxing breath breaks frequently throughout the day to reduce tension.

A common sleep disturbance is waking each other up. It may be difficult for you to get used to sleeping in the same bed again. Some couples handle the problem by sleeping separately. Unless this is absolutely necessary, I caution against it, as it may become a permanent barrier to sleeping together. Once one of you has moved to a separate bed or another bedroom, it may be difficult to find a reason to return. The time apart may create feelings of shyness or a reluctance to ask for the physical closeness you need.

Deciding who will shop for the low-sodium items at the supermarket may be easier than expressing your need to be cuddled and held. But physical touching is very important. Just as food preparation can be a vehicle to express love, sharing the same bed is an opportunity for intimacy.

For the sake of your rest and in order to preserve your closeness, talk with your mate about the issues of sleep. Remember; you, too, have been through a crisis. It takes rest and care for *your* body and *your* heart to heal.

SLEEPING HINTS

- Give yourself permission to nap during the day.
- Take the phone off the hook when you rest.
- Consider earplugs to protect your sleep from your mate's restlessness.
- Don't rely on medication for sleep or relaxation.
- Let go of your expectations about adequate sleep
- Don't count the minutes and hours that you sleep; let how you feel be your guide.
- Listen to quiet music before going to bed.
- Drink something warm and soothing (and decaffeinated) in the evening.

Working Out Work

Many of you are dealing with your spouse's sudden or early retirement. Some heart patients are recommended to change jobs to something less physically or psychologically demanding. Others may need to work fewer hours. Nothing changes things more quickly in a family-owned business than to have the boss suddenly hit with a cardiac problem.[2] Yet eighty-five percent of surviving heart attack victims are physically able to return to normal activity within three to six months after returning home.

During the early weeks of recuperation, no one knows how complete recovery will be.

I remember worrying incessantly about whether Marsh would be able to go back to work as a full-time architect. It was excruciating to wait, not knowing if he would be permanently disabled or handicapped by angina. Most of all, I worried about the uncertainty of our future. I felt especially anxious about our financial responsibilities, because we still had two adolescents at home. Like most heart attack survivors, Marsh was fortunate to be able to return to his work after six weeks, at first for four hours a day, and eventually full time.

I have worked with cardiac spouses who were less fortunate. Claudia and Peter, both in their mid-fifties, were told after Peter's bypass surgery that he should change jobs. Selling real estate was too stressful. Before Peter's surgery, Claudia's salary had been only supplemental. Her night job as a nurse's aide now became their sole source of income. As they watched their life savings dwindle, Peter and Claudia began to feel scared and depressed. Finally they sought professional help. In order to qualify for vocational training, Peter was classified as "disabled" by the state. He was trained in a government rehabilitation program and, after a full year of unemployment, finally found a job. No one addressed what that stigma had meant to him, just as earlier, no one had considered the stress he would undergo being unemployed. Six months later, Claudia became ill and needed to have fibroid tumor surgery. Her strength through the cardiac crisis and the year of Peter's unemployment, her stability as a breadwinner and wife, had taken their toll. She became the patient and needed to be cared for.

Whether your spouse retires, changes vocation, or stays with the same job, it's important for you to be involved in making the decisions. You may hesitate to express your opinion because you don't want to add any stress. But the stress already exists. Your questions and concerns are probably very similar to your mate's.

It is *normal and stressful* for a heart patient to be concerned about what recovery really means. He asks himself any number of questions: Will pain prohibit my normal activity? Will reduced cardiac efficiency keep me from working at my regular pace? Will I have to change jobs? Will my wife respect me if I can no longer be the breadwinner? Will we be able to pay the bills with less income? What kind of sacrifices will we have to make? Discussing these issues can reduce the burden each of you is carrying alone. Together you may be able to devise a more creative plan to cope with the financial distress and the work situation. Two heads are better than one, and being supportive of each other's recovery will yield benefits to both.

Economic pressures are only one aspect of work stress during recovery. Returning to work creates new tensions. Employers may under- or over-estimate how long your mate needs to shift gears. Fellow workers may want to discuss your spouse's cardiac experience when your spouse wants to forget that it happened. Or conversely, colleagues may be uncomfortable talking about heart disease and avoid your mate's need to talk.

You may be involved in your own career as well as trying to facilitate your mate's recovery. It may be necessary for you to make adjustments in your work schedule or even to change jobs in order to provide for your family.

One of the hardest lessons I learned as a cardiac spouse was the importance of going on with my own life. I had to alter my work schedule to account for the changes that were happening in my personal life. At times I was too distraught to give my full attention to my therapy clients. There were days when I felt guilty for being healthy, going off to work, and leaving Marsh at home alone. I felt uncomfortable sharing my enthusiasm and sense of accomplishment about work because I thought Marsh might feel envious or anxious about his own career. At other times, work was a refuge, a place where I didn't think about myself and I could focus on someone else. I needed to return to my work because it gave me stability and a sense of normalcy. It also helped to reduce my anxiety about our finances.

In some cases, cardiac spouses sacrifice their own careers because of their mate's heart disease. When Marjorie first came to see me, she complained of boredom. As a young, single parent, she had developed a successful management career and had raised her three children. She recalled her loneliness during those years, but her responsibilities to her children had kept her working hard, and her career success was a source of great satisfaction. She considered herself a valuable member of society.

Once her children were grown and her responsibilities reduced, she began to see Phillip, a business colleague. Although he was ten years older, they decided to marry. She had the best of both worlds: a stimulating career and a husband who was a close companion and an equal in business.

After four wonderful years together, Phillip had a seriously damaging heart attack. Marjorie decided to retire with him, although she was only fifty-three at the time. Since his cardiac crisis, Phillip and Marjorie have been inseparable. The only time they are apart is once a week, when a friend comes to take Phillip out for lunch. Marjorie misses the stimulation of her job and her old way of life. Honoring her marriage at the expense of her career, Marjorie has sacrificed an important aspect of her identity and her self-esteem. Now she is looking for something that will give her own life a broader meaning. But a lifestyle change is not so simple. Phillip relies heavily on her for care, attention, and security. She feels responsible for his health and worries about what will happen if there is another emergency and she is gone. She needs to find ways to give her own life meaning without jeopardizing her marriage.

Coping with work changes can be extremely stressful for both of you. There is no one right answer for any cardiac couple. It is important to discuss work issues. Avoiding them won't make them disappear. Ignoring such a sensitive topic may become the biggest problem of all. Seek professional counsel if you and your mate cannot talk about your feelings.

Discussions about work can be practical and productive. You may discover that your feelings are similar. Each of you is learning to make adjustments and redefine priorities. Once you can talk, you can brainstorm about your options. Perhaps together you can devise a plan of flexible re-entry into the work force. You may be able to use each other as a reality check. Does retirement really mean reduced social activity? Are younger people avoiding you or are you slowing down? Where will you find mental stimulation and meaning if you retire now? What does retirement mean to each of you?

Maybe you will find some useful projects around the house to complete during recuperation. If you talk about your mutual concerns, this recovery period can also be a time to get reacquainted as a couple, and to begin long-term planning based on your realistic appraisal of possibilities and new priorities. Sharing your concerns may ease your fears, diminish your loneliness, and allow you to work as a team.

Simple Pleasures

Obviously, your social and leisure activities have been affected by the "cardiac life-style." What before seemed like simple decisions - whether to go to a movie or play doubles tennis - become major issues in adjusting to a heart-healthy life. You want to protect your mate's health, but at the same time maintain your friendships and other interests.

When I first met Loreen, a thirty-seven-year-old cardiac spouse, she was trying to cope with changes in her social life. Six weeks after Tony's heart attack, Loreen planned a celebration barbecue for some of their friends. It was a beautiful summer evening. Everyone enjoyed the company, the good food, the new deck, and the lovely yard. Loreen felt pleased with her party and grateful that her life, so recently in chaos, was back to normal. She glanced at Tony and found him fast asleep in the lawn chair. It wasn't even dark yet! And what about their guests?

Loreen talked about how she felt that night: lonely,

embarrassed, angry, and sad. She also shared her worries about her future. What other life-style limitations would she encounter? How would she control her resentment if, at thirty-seven, her social life were to be permanently restricted?

Loreen's questions are not hers alone. Many cardiac spouses wonder the same things, especially during the active recovery stage (the first three months after a heart attack or a procedure), as the cardiac patient regains strength through a combination of rest and graduated activity. It is not unusual for a cardiac patient to nod off occasionally, even when something interesting is happening. You may feel embarrassed or impatient if your mate drifts in and out of conversation or moves at a snail's pace. You may question his motivation or even harbor resentment that he isn't improving more quickly. You may need to alter your expectations during recovery. The cardiac patient needs time and psychological space to integrate the many changes resulting from heart disease.

There isn't anything you can do to speed up the process. However, there are ways to adapt to it. During this period, you may ask your friends to be more flexible in accommodating themselves to your needs. It is likely that they will be understanding and tolerant of the situation. A rigorous night at the bowling alley may be replaced by a quiet evening watching VCR movies and munching salt-free popcorn.

As the weeks go by and your spouse's physical recovery progresses, you may wonder when it's appropriate to return to your hobbies, avocational activities, and friendships. At what point is it okay to resume your weekly tennis game, luncheon out with friends, an evening bridge game, volunteer work, the monthly book club meeting, or other activities you were involved in before? You may feel guilty going out and enjoying yourself when your part-

ner is home in bed. Or you may think that the seriousness of heart disease precludes recreation and fun. Some
cardiac spouses are afraid of criticism, worrying that being seen in public "having a good time" when a spouse
has suffered a heart attack implies that they are insensitive, uncaring, or selfish. Others just don't feel the old
enthusiasm for projects that had been important before
all this began.

The decision to resume your own activities is an
individual matter. It's very important to be involved in
something besides caring for your recovering mate. Time
for yourself, whether it's reading a book, exercising, or
shopping with a friend, is an important part of this transition. Maintaining interests in other areas of your life is
essential for your own needs and to restore a realistic
balance to your relationship.

Every cardiac couple is different when it comes to
the level of expectation for social and leisure activities.
However, you can realistically expect your mate to make
gradual progress and to have more energy each week.

There is the possibility that your mate sustained
substantial heart damage that will permanently restrict
his physical activity. You may be a marathon runner, or
just a weekend jogger, but your mate may now find it difficult to walk a flight of stairs or get through dinner without being short of breath.

Some cardiac spouses give up their own physical
activities to reduce the differences and avoid conflict.
Others change their activities temporarily or adjust their
paces to match their mates'. If you are feeling uncomfortable about exercising when it isn't an option for your partner, be sure to talk about it together. Assess your physical health and emotional well-being before making a decision based only on your spouse's condition and prognosis. Keep in mind that your choices may be short-term

and that your mate's condition will continue to change.

The cardiac life-style doesn't require you to trade in your running shoes for a cane and a pair of bifocals. Set the old bedridden stereotype aside. Recent medical trends have stressed the importance of regular exercise to strengthen the cardiovascular system and the general health of the heart patient. If your spouse participates in a cardiac rehabilitation program, he will get the supervised exercise he needs as well as a support network of fellow patients.

Recovery programs usually encourage cardiac spouses to participate. Regular exercise is important for *your* physical health, too. I recommend it as an antidote for restless nights, irregular appetite, and general lack of energy. Exercise is also an activity that the two of you may enjoy doing together.

Adding regular exercise to your routine requires effort, but it will more easily become a part of your schedule if you plan physical activity together three or four times a week. Whether you walk, bike, swim, or exercise more strenuously, what's important for health is to exercise regularly. Of course, you should check any exercise plan with your doctor before you begin. And doing something special together is another opportunity for closeness and companionship.

On The Road Again

Visiting and vacationing are a natural way of life for we mobile North Americans: jumping into the car, heading away for the weekend - to a cabin, the shore, the mountains, the kids' house to see the grandkids' newest feats.

Yet once heart disease enters the picture, what was

normal feels monumental. Vacation times, once eagerly anticipated and planned for, are fraught with fears and concerns. For most heart patients and heartmates, there are no restrictions placed on travel once early months of recovery are past. Doctors haven't limited travel, but many heartmates feel the danger of travel, the anxiety of uncertainty.

Cardiac spouses respond uniquely to the issue of travel. Derek expressed fear: "I'm too scared to go on vacation away from her doctor and hospital." Harriet said, "His heart attack happened away from home on a business trip. It was so hard there, away from family and friends. I never want to travel again." Shelley had a very different reaction: "My heart is broken. We used to spend a weekend a month driving down to see our grandchildren. It's been four months since his surgery and he refuses to travel and won't even tell me why." And finally Pam, "I feel so cheated. We always said that when we got to this age, we would see all the places we dreamed of. I feel guilty because I blame him for getting sick, for being so involved in his own health and not even noticing my desire to travel. What can I do with my get-up-and-go energy? How can I stop resenting him and heart disease?"

When your normal routines change, whether by choice or circumstances beyond your control, your stress increases. Your anxiety button gets pushed, probably because anything out of the ordinary automatically triggers the memory of your mate's cardiac event, and anxiety is not far behind.

Since that unexpected moment, you have used much of your energy to keep everything orderly and safe. Wanting to travel brings you face to face with a paradox. You want everything to stay under control, safe and secure, unchanged. But by its very nature, travel is a break from routine. A trip can be a wonderful change, offering new sights to see, new people to meet, new experiences to savor, and new learning.

Setting your mind at ease will allow you to enjoy your trip more fully. Understanding your discomfort with the unexpected is the first step in planning your next trip. Share the planning and responsibilities with your mate to ensure that you have a successful trip.

THE HEARTMATES® PACKING LIST

Your doctor and professional staff can provide answers to many of your questions about travel. Call the office for clarification about travel limitations including:

- Destination. Heart patients may need to avoid high altitudes such as the Rocky Mountains, Alps, or Andes. Higher altitudes have a lower oxygen level, and lack of oxygen places greater stress on the heart. Air quality in China is poor.
- To see if it's okay to mix heart medications with common travel medications for air or sea sickness, stomach upsets, diarrhea, etc.
- For referral to a physician or health facility in the city you plan to visit.
- To get a copy of your mate's most recent cardiogram and history to carry in your wallet or purse. Your doctor's office staff can make this available by using a simple copying machine.
- For any specific cautions your doctor might have for your mate. Have those clearly stated and agreed to between you and your spouse before you leave home.
- Carry a duplicate set of medications in a separate place for the duration of your trip. Always travel with medications in your carry-on luggage and/or purse. Have a

complete set of prescriptions with you as a secondary precaution.

- Make a habit of checking emergency medical procedures when you check-in to the hotel just as you would check the fire evacuation plan and exits from your room. If 911 isn't used, familiarize yourself with the procedure to get emergency help.
- Buy or rent a cellular phone for automobile trips so that access to emergency help is only 911 away. Be sure to provide family members with the cellular phone num ber.
- If you plan to travel outside the country, contact the embassy or consulate there for a list of English-speaking doctors. Phone numbers for embassies and consu lates are available through your local library, many travel books, your travel agent, or travel service.
- Check with your insurance agent for the availability of special emergency or evacuation insurance for out-of-country travel.

Doing some of these simple things will reduce your fear so you can enjoy the excitement, the fun, and the stimulation of travel. Feeling prepared, you can hit the road ready to enjoy yourself. When you discover a surprise, take a deep breath and remind yourself that you and your mate are okay and well prepared. Have a great time!

Who Are You Now? A Question Of Identity

You can change the way you cook, and you can adjust to coming home earlier on Saturday night. You can exercise regularly, and you can learn to live with less money, and you will still be you. But the changes that cardiac spouses experience go deeper. They affect the very center of your identity.

Identity is often experienced in the roles you play in daily life. People commonly identify themselves according to their responsibilities, by what they do, not who they are. For example, I would describe my primary roles as wife, mother, sister, friend, therapist, daughter, and writer. In addition, your identity is dictated by your beliefs about the world. If you say you are an optimist, a "people" person, or a devout Christian, you are identifying yourself in another way.

As a cardiac spouse, your roles and your beliefs are in the process of changing. From the first moment of the cardiac crisis, when you were faced with all those new responsibilities, you assumed a different type of behavior. While continuing to maintain your regular activities, you took charge of healthy meal planning, medication schedules, visiting hours, and keeping your family intact.

Since a cardiac crisis happens quickly and requires immediate action, it is natural to step into new roles without even noticing you're doing so.[3] But if you stop to look, you might be surprised to see that you have taken on one or more of the following roles.

THE HEAD NURSE

- Does your everyday vocabulary include words like pulse rate, angina, edema, stress test?
- Have you become an expert on the side effects of medications?
- Are you constantly adding questions to your list for your next call to the doctor?
- Is it difficult for you to go "off duty" and just relax with your mate?

If this sounds familiar, you may be wearing the crisp starched cap and white uniform of the Head Nurse. Although your patient load is light, it really matters. Keeping track of medications and communicating with the doctor may seem to be your official duties. Even though you don't have any medical training, you feel fully responsible for your mate's recovery. Also, it may be reassuring to take on the nurse's role, because the duties are so clearly defined. However, it can be very exhausting to feel as if your mate's health depends on your constant medical supervision. Even though there are pill bottles everywhere, your home is still your home, not a hospital. You are needed as a helpmate, not as a nurse.

THE TRAFFIC COP

- Are you constantly on guard for danger?
- Do you check to see if each medication is taken on time?
- Do you pride yourself on your ability to make fast decisions?
- Are the words "slow down" always on the tip of your tongue?

It is perfectly natural for you to want to take charge, to want to replace chaos with order. There are schedules to be followed and decisions to be made. It's important to take your responsibilities seriously. Heart disease is no laughing matter. However, it isn't necessary to acquire the stiff-brimmed hat and dress blues of the Traffic Cop. Your well-meaning efforts to keep your mate's recovery on track may have included taking an authoritative stance. It's stressful for you to be on guard all the time. And your mate may interpret your concern as control rather than support. Perhaps it's time to turn in your uniform and whistle. Guiding, not directing, traffic will be better for both of you.

THE CHEF

- Have you purchased more than two new cookbooks in search of heart-healthy recipes?
- Do you feel discouraged when your mate doesn't compliment you on your culinary skills?
- Do you insist on bringing your mate's own meal from home when you are invited to someone's house for dinner?
- Do you spend hours reading nutritional charts?

If creating heart-healthy meals has become your full-time career, you may have slipped into the role of the Chef. You constantly look for healthy, delectable recipes, hoping to aid your mate's recovery and elevate his spirits. Being the Chef is a way for you to feel positively involved in improving your mate's health. However, you might feel let down if, after slaving away in the kitchen, he doesn't appear to appreciate your efforts. If you take off your white toque and apron, you will be less likely to set yourself up for disappointment. Cardiac patients often aren't enthusiastic about eating. Your mate's appetite is not a reflection of your culinary ability or of his love.

THE MOTHER

- Do you find yourself constantly worrying, wringing your hands, pacing back and forth?
- Do you find yourself talking to your mate in a soothing and pacifying tone?

• Is all of your attention devoted to your mate's care?
• Are you afraid to leave your home in case your mate needs your help?

When someone you love hurts, it is natural to feel protective. But if most of your time is spent coddling and taking care of your mate, you may have unknowingly taken on the role of the Mother. Mothers are known for their nonstop worrying and selfless giving. It's one reason why they're always so tired. Right now it may be necessary to do more than your usual share. But if you have a perpetually worried look on your face, you may be taking on more responsibility than is good for either of you. Treating your spouse like a youngster will only add to his feelings of helplessness. And after a while, you may begin to resent his demands. Your mate needs your help, but he doesn't need you to be his mother. And you don't need another child.

Coping with Change

As you can see by looking at all the stereotypes described above, much more than your life-style has been changed by the cardiac crisis. You may not be aware of how much your roles and identity have changed. Most people find it difficult to be objective about themselves.

This evaluation guide will help you assess the changes in your life. Many cardiac spouses have found it valuable to write their responses in a Heartmates® notebook or journal. Writing clarifies thinking; it is a safe way to express feelings and is a useful reference during later stages of recovery. Major categories of change, such as food, are listed. Following each category are guidelines to help you explore specific changes within the category. Consider each aspect as it relates to your life before and after the cardiac crisis.

HEARTMATES® ASSESSMENT OF CHANGE

Sleep

Quantity
Quality
Disturbances
Dreams and nightmares
Frequency of naps

Food

Level of appetite
Time spent shopping
Time spent preparing food
Frequency of eating out
Primary foods
Priority in your life

Exercise

Type
Frequency
Quantity
Strenuousness
Regularity
Differences between you

Leisure Activities

Types of involvemen
Schedule and hours
Level of satisfaction
Quality of work

Financial Responsibilities

Providing income
Budgeting
Allocating funds
Handling banking

Work/Career

Degree of involvement
Schedule and hours
Level of satisfaction
Quality of work

Friends/Social Activities

Frequency
Quality of time spent
Level of satisfaction
Initiating activity

Once you have an objective sense of the changes that have already occurred, you can begin to understand those with which you are satisfied and where you want to initiate further change. For example, if you notice that you have let a friendship lapse, invite someone over or plan an outing with a friend. You have the power to reach out for the support and understanding that you need. On the other hand, you may be very pleased with the modifications you've made in your diet. Your spouse's cardiac condition may have caused you to focus attention on your own physical health and your need to eat differently.

Given the unexpectedness of the cardiac crisis and the pace at which you have functioned during your partner's recovery, it may be a real relief to stop and take stock. The ability to step back and look is a good sign that you are on the road to recovery.

It may be difficult to go over financial papers, wills, and insurance, because it acknowledges mortality. But once you have done this, you may find a sense of peace replacing the panic in your chest. Your nightmare of having to sell all your possessions will be replaced by a more realistic assessment of your earning skills. Facing your fiscal reality increases your trust in your own resilience and flexibility. If you've always left the finances to your mate, pretending you don't have a head for figures, then assuming more responsibility might increase your confidence in yourself. You might even find that you like doing the family accounting.

An essential first step in coping with change is comprehending what has happened to you, by taking an objective look at yourself and your situation. The next step is to acknowledge your strengths in dealing with the crisis thus far. It's important to recognize that you have managed to the best of your ability through a difficult time.

It isn't easy to affirm your strengths. Most of us are more comfortable with criticism than with compliments. We find it difficult to appreciate our positive qualities, and we are more aware of our weaknesses than of our strengths. You may even be admonishing yourself with internal dialogue — "I should be more caring and attentive. . . I should be more worried about him . . . I shouldn't relax my vigil. . . I shouldn't feel bad, sad, or mad. . . I shouldn't have a good time or enjoy myself." And, above all, "I don't deserve to give myself any credit for handling the cardiac crisis well, because I haven't done it perfectly."

No one is perfect! But taking credit for doing your best is an important part of the recovery process. Something that has worked well for many cardiac couples is making a pact to share one thing each day that you appreciate about yourselves. In that way a realistic and ongoing assessment of your situation can continue. You will have something worthwhile to talk about with each other every day.

Continued assessment of the ongoing changes will help you recognize and accept reality. I would like to be able to tell you that the road to recovery is straight and narrow, but I know that it rarely is. The road sign reads "Uncertainty," and accepting that requires a new belief in your ability to live with permanent change. For many cardiac spouses, the most difficult part of aftercare is coming to terms with uncertainty. The road is different for every cardiac spouse. For some, the road may have more potholes and unexpected turns. If you are fortunate, recovery may be a long, lasting journey, and the reality of a life with someone with heart disease may be accepted as simply part of growing older together.

CHAPTER NOTES

1. One of my favorite cardiac cookbooks is *Craig Claiborne's Gourmet Diet*, written by Craig Claiborne with Pierre Franey (New York: Ballantine Books, 1980.) It includes low-sodium and modified-cholesterol recipes. Our favorite recipe is the Lemon Chicken, Texas style. See also more recent and very useful books by Joseph C. Piscatella, of the Institute for Fitness and Health: *The Fat Tooth Fat Gram Counter*, and *Restaurant & Fast Food Fat-Gram Counter*, and his earlier *The Don't Eat Your Heart Out Cookbook ; Controlling Your Fat Tooth;* and *Choices for a Healthy Heart.*

2. When the owner of a family business has a cardiac crisis, two basic steps need to be implemented: planning about leadership and sharing the plan with everyone involved. Professionals who specialize in guiding families who want to insure the continuity of their family business are available. One such resource is McGladrey & Pullen, a firm nationally recognized for their work with families in family business. Contact Steve Swartz at (612) 376-9346 in McGladrey & Pullen's Minneapolis office.

3. Dona Wilson is the cardiac spouse program facilitator (in cardiac rehabilitation) in Carson City, Nevada. Dona collected hats designating the roles described here. After picking a hat from her basket and trying it on, each spouse read the description of the matching role from this chapter. This technique allowed spouses to experience the roles that went with each hat without guilt, and animated discussion followed. If you have an idea you found useful in your recovery that you'd like to share, please write us at P.O. Box 16202, Mpls., MN 55416 or use our e-mail address: Heartmates@aol.com or on the WorldWideWeb: http://www.heartmates.com/

3

At The Heart Of The Matter

I recently encountered a woman whose husband had just passed his six-month mark. I congratulated her on his recovery. She nodded thanks, but something about her expression made me wonder if she was okay. When I gently asked her, she recounted a familiar story. Ever since her husband's return from the hospital, their marriage had become increasingly stressful. Before his surgery they had been compatible and close. Now they vacillated between constant bickering and strained silence. Their home, which had always been a haven, was beginning to seem like a battleground.

This woman's story reminded me of how difficult a marriage relationship can be in the first six to twelve months of recovery. Paradoxically, there is much to be thankful for. You feel grateful beyond measure that your mate has recovered, regained strength, and is back on his feet. The image of him weak and vulnerable in the hospital is slowly fading. It's not so easy to recall fitful sleep and irregular meals, or the sense of disorientation and helplessness. You've probably acquired enough expertise about medications, diet, and the terminology that accompanies cardiac disease to run the educational program at the hospital. Your husband has not called a doctor in weeks, maybe even months.

It's a relief to settle back into a regular routine. The new order, incorporating scheduled exercise and dietary changes, is almost second nature. There is less pressure on you to care for a patient, and you have enough time for family, activities, and work. Friends and relatives have returned to their normal lives, and don't call or visit as often. Some days you don't even react when you get an unexpected telephone call or hear an ambulance siren in the night.

And yet *your* transition continues. You looked forward to celebrating your mate's recovery. Some days you feel great; other days you can't seem to pull yourself out of the doldrums. Your spouse has returned to work and your family is "back to normal." *But what was normal before bears little or no resemblance to life as you know it today.*

Your life is different. There are a number of issues that make this period especially complicated. The one person you normally count on for support is emotionally out of reach. Ironically, your mate may be around more, but you feel lonelier than ever.[1] Heart patients are, as a rule, engrossed in their physical symptoms. Even when your spouse is physically present, his preoccupation with himself may leave little room for your needs.

Your mate may also be more demanding of your time and want you to stay nearby just for security. Activities that you used to share, like volunteer work or playing in a mixed bowling league, may no longer interest your partner or may be out of the question because of medical limitations. If your routine keeps you at home with your recovering spouse, the increased proximity may limit your mobility and freedom. You may even begin to feel smothered, as if you are losing yourself in this entity called heart disease.

Your relationship with your spouse has changed in both obvious and subtle ways. No one has a perfect marriage. But you probably consider your spouse one of the half dozen people you are closest to in the world. Before the cardiac crisis you may have told your mate about things that were important to you. You probably discussed opinions and issues on a regular basis. You may have shared inner secrets, hopes, and dreams. At times, you experienced regular physical closeness and sexual intimacy. You felt a connection partially made up of years spent together ... living, working, and raising a family.

The onset of the cardiac crisis caused a major break in your relationship. First, there was the physical separation; you slept at home while your mate, surrounded by medical equipment and strangers, slept in the hospital. Then, there was a breakdown in communications. The shock of the crisis made you unsure of what to say or how to respond. You got the message that your spouse needed rest and shouldn't experience stress. You wore makeup to cover the dark circles under your eyes, a product of stress and sleeplessness, and you were the cheerleader who encouraged him on the short, slow walk down the hospital corridor. You tried to act cheerful and upbeat when you really felt worried and sad. You held back your tears so that he wouldn't be burdened by your anguish. The more you disguised your feelings, the greater the distance grew between you.

For some couples, there is a carry-over of that emotional distance into the recovery phase and beyond. You may still be as withdrawn as you were when you stood at his hospital bedside. Your communication with each other may be stilted for fear of creating stress or making each other feel worse. You may even believe that your relationship is so fragile that it will begin to fall apart if you start talking.

You may not be aware of the energy it takes to hide your feelings from your mate. And, in the long run, you are setting up a mode of communication that inhibits rather than promotes honesty in your marriage. Your partner may wonder what really lies beneath your cheerful countenance, or resent your apparent confidence when he is feeling so scared. Besides, he needs to be needed now, too. Why not break down the barriers by reaching out to each other? There is an old adage that goes: When you share joy it is doubled; when you share pain it is halved.

Those Powerful Feelings

Feelings are your reaction to the world around you. Your feelings are the normal and predictable responses to the cardiac crisis you have experienced. You need to acknowledge and respect them as real and important.

It's natural to put off dealing with your feelings in the height of the emergency. But the emergency is over! And your feelings have not disappeared. In fact, some of them are stronger. It is harder to ignore and control them as the weeks and months pass. They get in the way and intensify what is already a difficult situation between you and your mate. Trying to control your feelings takes a great deal of energy, and may strain your relationship with your mate beyond the original crisis.

Though he may not have expressed it verbally, your spouse is struggling with similar feelings. Most of the professional attention he received concentrated on his physical care. Friends focus their encouragement on tangible aspects of recovery like improved endurance and increased strength. But the depth of the emotional, mental, and spiritual crisis the cardiac patient weathers is often unrecognized.

Remember your spouse has to make emotional adjustments while he copes with the physical realities of heart disease. Most likely, it is a struggle for him to accept what has happened. Facing physical limitations, heart patients are prone to volatile feelings. Some patients manifest their anger by being demanding, withdrawn, irritable, or overly solicitous. Others demonstrate their fear by denying that anything has changed. They may act out by continuing to smoke and eat the wrong foods. They may lift heavy objects, return to work without permission from their physician, or push physical limits until they're exhausted. One woman insisted on vacuuming and scrubbing her kitchen floor one month after bypass surgery. She admitted to being independent and stubborn. But she was also unwilling to limit herself or care wisely for herself, even before her incision pain had disappeared.

Most of us find it difficult to step into another person's emotional shoes. When you are in the midst of an intense experience, you cannot readily identify and empathize with anyone else's feelings. But you ought to try to understand what your mate is going through for two reasons: so you can see how his attitude and behavior are affecting you, and so you can begin to support each other. Your spouse's physical heart has healed, and you need not fear damaging it by stating your feelings and concerns.

Feelings can be divided into two general categories: positive and negative, experienced as pleasurable and painful. When you experience a crisis, you suffer an emotional wound. It's common for people to try to avoid or ignore the resulting painful feelings. When something happens that is beyond personal control, people move unconsciously to what is familiar. The most common reaction is to fall back on habitual behavior.

Most of us like to think of ourselves as kind, open, and loving. We find it more difficult to accept our anger and disappointment. Guilt, fear, and sadness may be more familiar, but they can be overwhelming. All of these feelings are appropriate responses to the intense changes you have experienced. If you're like most cardiac spouses, you may have thought, or even voiced, something like: "I'm trying to do everything right, but I can't stop crying. . . I'm snapping at everyone all the time. . . It's so hard to keep my hopes up when I'm so worried. . . I'm afraid I'm coming apart, and I don't know what to do about it. . . Why do I feel depressed when he is recovering so well?"

All of these feelings are normal. Give yourself permission to have all of your feelings, including the "negative" ones, and you will be more able to do something about them. The first step is to recognize what they are.

Anxiety, the Great Paralyzer

Cardiac spouses experience profound fears. What are they, and why are they so powerful? You have been thrown abruptly into a situation that threatens all aspects of your life. Once the initial terror passes, you are faced with the great unknown. Before the cardiac crisis you felt relatively secure and sure of yourself. Now you feel anxious and uncertain about the future.

Anxiety is defined as the fear of being hurt or losing something. All cardiac spouses are afraid of losing their partners. This kind of fear manifests itself in thinking of foreboding questions without any answers. During the interminable hours you waited outside the hospital emergency room, wondering whether your mate was still alive, close to death, resting comfortably, or in excruciating pain, you undoubtedly asked yourself: Will my mate survive? Perhaps your anxiety was most acute at the beginning of the crisis, when everything was touch and go. Or perhaps your numbness might have protected you, whereas now you are haunted by questions of survival. In either case, the terrible fear of being widowed doesn't evaporate the minute your mate is discharged from the hospital. Surgical success and cardiac rehabilitation aside, no heart patient is given a clean bill of health. Consequently, all cardiac spouses live with the anticipation and fear of a fatal episode. Your anxiety can be provoked quickly and easily. Think about how you feel when your spouse cuts your regular walk short without telling you why. Consider your reaction when you see him "popping nitros," checking his pulse, or taking his blood pressure.

Emily was called long distance and informed that her husband had suffered a heart attack. He was in a strange city, halfway across the country, where he was attending a sales show. Emily and Theo had no family in their city to take care of their two young daughters, but Emily quickly made emergency arrangements with a friend, and flew off to support and help care for Theo.

Terrified and alone in a motel in a strange city, Emily had to rely on the advice of strangers. She slept poorly, ate hurriedly in coffee shops, and spent as much time as she could with Theo in a strange hospital.

It was frightening, lonely, and stressful to spend each day in the hospital and to return to a motel room each night. Having to function as an optimistic messenger for Theo's worried parents and their own frightened children, Emily quickly exhausted much of her energy. As Theo's recovery progressed, a nurse gave Emily explicit instructions about getting him home safely, and caring for him once there. She advised purchasing first-class seats on the airplane, and arranging for wheelchair support at the airport to meet Theo at the gate when they arrived.

Finally they were on their way home. Just before landing, the flight attendant came over to them, leaned toward Theo, and said, "The wheelchair for your wife is at the gate, so don't worry." Emily's fear had taken so great a toll that she was mistaken for the cardiac patient who needed special care.

The fear of losing your mate escalates if he doesn't seem committed to recovery. His seemingly cavalier attitude may frustrate you. You simply don't trust his good judgment about how much he can do. Anxiety mounts as you see that your mate hasn't stopped smoking or that he is gaining weight. How can you help but panic when he insists on shoveling snow, moving furniture, lifting heavy boxes, or jogging too far? It isn't unusual for heart patients to test their limits, to prove something to themselves or to feel useful and needed. Men may feel added pressure to reassert their masculinity. Whatever the reason, it adds up to more anxiety for you.

Most people experience anxiety as a combination of physical symptoms mixed with an overwhelming sense of helplessness. In cases of severe anxiety, you may feel unsettled, agitated, or frantic. Your heartbeat may speed up and butterflies may flutter in your stomach. You may shake or tremble uncontrollably, sweat, get cold feet and hands. Less intense reactions include tense muscles, tightening of neck and shoulders, clenched teeth, and a vague sense of impending loss.

I remember the terror. It began about the time Marsh was due to leave the hospital. I was terrified that he would die at any moment now that we were away from the doctor and the nursing staff; terrified that he'd never recover enough to resume his place in the family as husband, father, and breadwinner; terrified that I wouldn't have the inner strength to care for him, to maintain my responsibilities as the new leader of the family. I was terrified that I felt so alone and no one seemed to know, and terrified that now that Marsh was home everyone would abandon us, believing we no longer needed their support or help. And, most of all, I was terrified that just thinking this way proved that I was crazy, abnormal, or that I had cracked under the pressure.

Another fear expressed by many cardiac spouses is that of being abandoned, being left alone. For a younger cardiac spouse it may evoke fears of inadequacy, of inability to raise children alone. But, for older cardiac spouses, whose children have grown and left home, the thought of being widowed can be even worse. Merriam, a seventy-year-old cardiac spouse, remarried late in life. After losing her first husband to heart disease, Merriam raised their two children alone. Once they were grown, she began to see an old high-school sweetheart, a widower. They married in their middle sixties, largely out of need for security and companionship. Merriam's second husband recently suffered a heart attack, and now Merriam has become terrified of abandonment. She finds it difficult to express her anxiety about aging and dying alone.

Since men experience heart disease earlier in life than most women, the majority of cardiac spouses are female. Older women are particularly vulnerable to financial survival fears, because a large percentage have worked exclusively as homemakers. Financial decisions are especially difficult during a time of crisis. Becoming a "bag lady" is a very real specter for many women. Others describe nightmares about the mortgage company appearing on the doorstep, threatening foreclosure.

Although I have worked for most of my adult years, I felt terrified about finances after Marsh's heart attack. My thinking, repetitious and negative, went something like this: "There's no way we can keep the house, we'll have to sell it. The kids have been so happy here. They'll hate living in a small apartment. There's probably not an apartment in this neighborhood that we can afford. The kids will have to change schools. How will I ever put them through college on my income alone?"

One morning, my terror escalated out of control. I called the social security office to ask how much money each of our children would get if Marsh died or was permanently disabled. Never mind that his heart attack had been described as minor by the doctor or that his recovery so far had been uncomplicated.

I was distraught. I needed information to calm me down, but then I struggled with another fear: Had I put a hex on Marsh's recovery? By thinking about money, disability, and death, I might have caused the very outcome I dreaded most, in a sort of self-fulfilling prophecy!

Seeking information is one coping strategy to help reduce anxiety. The more information you have, the fewer catastrophic fantasies you will imagine, and you will feel less out of control.

Chronic anxiety is common in situations where heart disease is severe and increasingly debilitating. When Edith first came to me, she needed help managing her overwhelming fears. Her husband, Richard, had suffered several heart attacks, bypass surgery, and almost every possible complication. Edith explained that she had called 911 numerous times over the last six years. She actively worried every time she left the house, dreading another emergency, convinced that she wouldn't be there to save him. Her stomach and head ached, her muscles were tight, her speech was clipped, and her movements were agitated and jumpy. She felt frantic each time she watched Richard take his pulse or heard him sigh audibly.

Edith was disappointed in herself because she couldn't control - or get rid of - her fear. She equated courage with fearlessness. When we talked about how strong she had been during the six years she cared for Richard, she said that fear had never stopped her from acting quickly or resolutely. And once Edith was able to appreciate her courage, she began to accept her fears.

When she hears Richard cough or sigh, Edith still experiences fear. But now, before her fears race ahead in her thoughts to a catastrophic conclusion, she takes a deep breath and says to herself, "I feel afraid and I have my courage." This helps her keep her fear from escalating, and reminds her of her strength.

The first step in dealing with anxiety is the hardest: You must admit that you are afraid. Fear is like an alarm that alerts us to defend and protect ourselves in a threatening situation. If you ignore your anxiety and pretend that everything is fine, you will spend energy you really can't afford and in no way alleviate your fear.

Once you recognize that you feel anxious, you need to ask yourself, "What am I afraid of losing?" Try to be very specific. Deal directly with the threat - do not ignore or deny it - and perceive your situation anew. You can then choose to accept what you cannot change, and plan ways to act on what you can change.

As you face your fears, it is equally important to take stock of your strengths, those qualities you can count on in yourself during an emergency or a difficult time. Look specifically at the cardiac crisis you have been through, and be sure to recognize what you have done well. View your strengths as an advantage in your plan to change what can be changed; they'll help you succeed.

People who have survived trauma, and cardiac spouses can be counted among them, are affected in a particular way. When you experience an unexpected and life-threatening event, your body instinctively goes into a survival mode. This gift of nature protects you during the cardiac crisis. But every change has its benefit and its cost. Because your chemical and physical body can't discriminate, you will automatically repeat the protective reaction every time you feel threatened. Your body is unable to differentiate between a life-threatening crisis and a less serious event. For example, you may find yourself as anxious when you find the toast burning in the toaster as you would if you found your house burning down.

When you experience a powerful reaction, you can oppose the automatic anxiety responses by doing three things:

1. Calm yourself down by focusing on taking deep breaths.
2 Share your thoughts and feelings with another person (there is no way to check reality in isolation).
3. Engage in positive self-talk (the goal is to be functional).

Why not ask a friend or relative to listen to your fears on a regular basis? Let your confidante know that you don't expect her to fix things, that what you need is an ear, and maybe a shoulder. Sometimes anxiety can be so severe or so prolonged that professional help, including anti-anxiety medication, is needed. Don't hesitate to consult your own physician if you find yourself unable to handle your anxiety.

Repeat the Serenity Prayer to yourself whenever you feel the need. It can be a powerful antidote to fear:

God,
grant me the serenity to
accept the things I cannot change,
the courage to change the things I can,
and the wisdom to know the difference.

The Ogre, Anger

Are you irritated, impatient, or resentful more frequently now than before the cardiac crisis? Do you find yourself yelling at no one in particular? Are you aggravated easily for no obvious reason? If so, you are experiencing feelings of anger, as do most cardiac spouses.

There are a variety of underlying reasons for your feelings of anger. Family and friends are likely to focus on the ailing cardiac patient, forgetting that you, too, are in a time of crisis. You may feel angry at the abundance of attention that your spouse receives. You certainly don't begrudge him that much-needed support, but it would be nice if occasionally someone recognized your needs.

Your anger may also be a mask for your fear or pain. Marie, a farm wife, reported her uncontrollable anger at her spouse. She explained that her cooking style, twenty-one meat and potato meals each week, had always been an accepted way to support the heavy farm work John did in the fields and barn ... until he had a heart attack. Marie learned a healthier style of cooking at the hospital. She planned meals and cooked the new way with the same gusto as she had before. For several months, she assured herself that she was doing the best possible thing for John; she had denied him fat in all the food she prepared. After supper one hot summer night, he drove off in his pickup truck. Twenty minutes later he returned with chocolate ice cream, which he ate ravenously with a large spoon directly from the carton.

Marie could not contain her anger, and shouted rageful things she didn't even know she thought: how hard she had worked to save his life by changing his diet, how inappreciative he was about her efforts, and that if he were going to commit suicide eating chocolate ice cream, she would just leave him. The next morning Marie could hardly believe those strong words had been hers. She was only aware of her fear that she would lose John.

You may feel angry at the professional team that cared for your spouse at the hospital, or be dissatisfied with the quality of services. One woman, a cardiac nurse by profession, was furious that certain drugs weren't administered to her husband. A receptionist who has put you on hold, a doctor in a hurry, or a distracted nurse who forgets to say hello are likely targets, even scapegoats, for your anger.

It is not unusual to feel angry or irrationally agitated about something as vague or abstract as heredity or genes. This is especially true if your spouse is a non-smoker who has been exercising and eating well for years. Some cardiac spouses resent their mates for having heart attacks and disrupting their lives. Others feel irritated at their spouses for not appearing to appreciate their efforts. Still others are angry at their partners for being insensitive to their feelings during this difficult time.

Josie, a cardiac spouse, described a family holiday scene. She, her husband, and their three young sons spent Thanksgiving with relatives. Even though Jack was scheduled to undergo bypass surgery the following Monday, Josie was determined to make the holiday as pleasant as possible. All afternoon members of the family crowded around Jack, asking how he was doing and giving him their best wishes. He was the star attraction, and most of the conversation centered around his illness and impending surgery. As the day wore on Josie became first irritated and then furious. She had desperately wanted Thanksgiving to be normal, especially for the sake of their children. She felt as if her life would never again be free from the focus on heart disease.

Cardiac spouses also feel angry because their own needs for support are sorely neglected. Everyone expresses concern for the patient. Rarely does anyone remember to ask about you. One man reported feeling like a newscaster responsible for giving up-to-the-minute reports on his wife's condition. One evening, after several such phone reports, he remembered thinking that if one more person called and asked, "How's Kathryn doing?" he would slam the phone down. He just needed someone to say, "How are *you* doing, Ken? I bet this is a really difficult time for you." Ken felt so angry that he was tempted to disconnect the phone. What he really needed was some warm, human connection for himself.

If you are accustomed to relying on your spouse to meet many of your emotional needs, your feelings of neglect may well be exacerbated. You're not getting the affection or support you need right now. You deeply miss your partner's interest in you, your daily activities, and your thoughts and ideas. Even if he was outgoing and openly affectionate before, he may now be self-centered and engrossed with his health. It seems that every time you look, he's checking his pulse, weighing himself, or taking his blood pressure. Despite your best efforts to sympathize and understand, you still feel angry at his apparent loss of interest in you and, possibly, his lack of appreciation.

So, where do you direct your feelings? Many cardiac spouses find it impossible to feel anger toward the patient. They unconsciously deny their anger out of loyalty, confusion, fear, or guilt. When this happens, that same anger may be transferred to the doctor, nursing staff, Fate, or even God. Or you may turn the anger inward, and berate yourself for not trying to make your husband quit smoking or stop working so hard.

Attempting to explain or justify your anger is fruitless. Feelings just aren't rational. Rationalizing them is like asking yourself if it is all right to be hungry or thirsty. Like hunger and thirst, feelings exist and are normal responses to your situation. You don't need to justify your feelings to yourself or to anyone else. Your anger is a signal that you are experiencing a crisis.

About anger, Stephanie Ericsson, author of *Companion Through The Darkness,* says it is "...our natural protective armor. It tells the rest of the world that a boundary has been violated. Our society would have us swallow it, and many of us do....Rage is white-hot anger....It is a superb emotion. Used correctly, it lays down permanent boundaries, stakes out lifetime territories, and gives us girth. It will launch us out of inertia and thrust us forward." [2] Use your anger energy to help you get your needs met.

Getting angry is *not* dangerous to your spouse's health. Of course, I'm not suggesting that you berate your mate during the first forty-eight hours after a heart attack. Nor do I advocate that you take advantage of the situation to act like a nasty ogre, spoiled brat, or a whining witch. Both you and your mate are experiencing angry feelings about all the changes that heart disease has created in your lives. Anger doesn't mean you don't love each other. You can find appropriate ways to express your anger and learn how to diffuse it, freeing yourself to move on.

There are many ways to express anger safely and appropriately. Some people release their anger physically.

You can pound the wall, swim laps vigorously, or smash a tennis or racquetball. Some people rid themselves of anger by writing. Yell into a pillow or shout in the shower - just raising your voice is a great release.

Direct communication is the most effective way to express anger to your mate. If this is threatening or unprecedented, begin by negotiating rules for the discussion. Rules provide safety and a foundation on which to build further communication.

- Set a time limit (five minutes may be sufficient) for each of you to speak.
- Name a place that is completely private.
- Make a pact that allows honest expression of anger.
- Agree not to interrupt.
- Commit to listening fully and openly.
- Take turns.
- Remember that you are on the same team and that you love each other.

Here is a list of "do's" and "don'ts" to help you express your anger.

HEARTMATES® ANGER CHECKLIST

DO	DON'T
Do say what hurts	Don't avoid talking about important issues
Do begin all angry statements with "I"	Don't use your anger to blame
Do use your anger to clear the air	Don't mistake anger for violence or aggression
Do try to make yourself understood	Don't exaggerate, whine, or complain
Do tell it straight	Don't rationalize or intellectualize
Do say what you think	Don't save up little irritations until your anger explodes
Do say regularly how you feel	Don't withdraw because you'll injure your mate
Do raise your voice until you're heard	Don't believe your relationship is too fragile to bear the weight of your feelings
Do take responsibility; "own" your anger	Don't sacrifice your anger in exchange for physical symtoms like headaches, depression, or ulcers
Do say you're angry	Don't use your anger attack or punish your mate

Sadness, the Heavy Weight

It may seem strange to feel sad at a time like this. Your mate is recovering. Shouldn't you be happy? Yes, but major life changes are also accompanied by feelings of sadness, even depression.

We all tend to take our lives for granted. When something happens that jeopardizes our security, we experience enormous feelings of loss. In a cardiac crisis, all that you hold near and dear has been threatened. The everyday freedom and long-term security you count on suddenly seems tenuous, or even lost.

You may recognize sadness or depression by its effects on your body. The physical counterparts sometimes appear as lethargy or fatigue. Cardiac spouses often attempt to hide their sadness for fear of appearing ungrateful, selfish, or spoiled. In the hospital and during the recovery period, you may have "put on a happy face," and worn a mask of cheerfulness and confidence.

As you relax your pose, you may become depressed. Symptoms of depression can creep up slowly, or hit you early and hard. Depression saps your energy and reduces your ability to function. For some time, you may feel as if nothing matters or that it takes all of your stamina just to get through the day. You may even begin to question the meaning and purpose of your life.

Janet, age thirty-nine, described her life before her husband's heart attack. She jokingly referred to herself as "the Tour Director." She was constantly organizing social activities for the two of them and their friends. They were enthusiastic sports fans and patrons of the repertory theater and local art museum. They made several business trips and took vacations each year. Making arrangements was almost a full-time job for Janet. Since Brendan's bypass surgery, Janet wanders through her immaculate condominium pondering the purpose of her life. The structure of her daily routine has toppled. Accustomed to organizing and taking charge, Janet feels lost, aimless, and adrift. She is wary of feeling sorry for herself because she has always felt so privileged. But her old life is gone. Her new life is still a question mark. The void leaves her feeling empty and confused.

Few cardiac spouses have lost such an exciting and romantic way of life, but all confront the disappointment of broken dreams. Margaret, a careful and conservative person, and her husband, Patrick, planned to realize a lifelong dream and retire to a quiet, rural town somewhere in a warm climate. Just one year before retiring from his construction job, Patrick suffered a severe heart attack. Their savings have dwindled because of medical and related expenses. Margaret empathizes with Patrick's fear and understands his need to stay in Wisconsin, where his doctor and family members can give him the support he needs. Still, she mourns the loss of her retirement cottage in the sun.

If your mate has a second heart attack or a setback during recovery that requires a procedure, both of you may feel more disappointed than you did at the onset of the cardiac crisis. Pamela's outlook was very positive when Jerry returned to work after recovering from his first heart attack. But she described her attitude after his second heart attack and surgery as negative, even despairing. She had a very hard time accepting his forced retirement when he was only fifty-three. Physical recovery may be more prolonged and your depression more difficult to overcome the second time around. It takes more effort to feel optimistic and to trust in the medications, in your recovery program, even in your doctor.

Some of the sadness that cardiac spouses report indicates yearning for things past: Christmas as it used to be when he dressed up like Santa to pass out gifts to the grandchildren; those few years comparatively free of responsibility after the children were grown and before her heart attack; long driving trips through the Northwest every summer until his cardiac surgery. Each holiday, every season marked from the onset of heart disease, is an occasion for gratitude *and* mourning.

I remember the audible sigh of relief when a cardiologist, speaking to a group of patients and spouses, acknowledged that it is *normal* for cardiac patients to experience depression. *The same is true for cardiac spouses and other cardiac family members.* In order to deal with depression, you must first acknowledge your sadness and disappointment. Facing your sadness may seem difficult and painful, even fearful. But disregarding it won't make it disappear. In fact, just the opposite is true. Once you accept that your feelings are legitimate, the terror will decrease. By allowing yourself to experience your sadness, you will gain faith in your resilience and confidence in your courage.

You need to let yourself grieve over your losses. This means mourning what *is* lost and can't be retrieved. It also means you must accept what is beyond your personal control. Mourning is a process, and you need to give yourself plenty of time to grieve. Don't feel that you have to be finished with your sadness or disappointment on anyone else's schedule. Don't be pressured by comments about "dwelling on your sadness" or implications that you should "hurry up and get on with your life."

One Sunday afternoon about two months after Marsh's heart attack, a friend called to invite me to the movies. It sounded like a perfect thing to do to get away. When it was time to get ready, I felt exhausted and won-

dered why I had agreed to the outing. I was surprised and disturbed to find that I could not keep my mind on the movie. Everyone in the theater laughed out loud, but I didn't find the clever repartee funny at all. I couldn't concentrate on or analyze the ideas presented in the film. Perhaps it was just too early for me to enjoy myself. But in the grand scheme of things, the movie seemed trivial in comparison with my personal struggles.

Our society supports quick decisions and avoidance of pain.[3] Remember that each individual is unique and experiences grief differently and at an individual pace. When Henry David Thoreau suggested that each person hears a different drummer and needs "to step to the music which he hears, however measured or far away,"[4] he might well have been honoring the recovery of the cardiac spouse.

You may be tempted to minimize or deny your own sadness on the pretense of sacrifice or good will, but it's a myth that "acting happy" will help your mate move through his depression more quickly. And it is absolutely not true that feeling bad is a sign of weakness, craziness, or failure. Expressing your sadness doesn't negate your feelings of gratitude that your mate is recovering. And, as the New Testament (Matthew 5:4) tells us, "Blessed are those who mourn, for they shall be comforted."

In time, your sadness will diminish. You'll know naturally when you've mourned enough. Your physical, emotional, and mental energy will return. You may suddenly feel motivated to do things that for months have seemed impossible. You will find yourself spontaneously interested in others again. Your focus will shift from yearning for a lost past to planning for your future.

The Grasp of Guilt

Guilt is a complicated feeling. Sometimes it is explained as anger turned in on yourself. It's no wonder so many cardiac spouses feel guilty. What kind of a woman would feel angry at a husband who's sick and almost died? But, again, feelings aren't rational, and your anger is real. With no one else to blame, you became angry at yourself.

Guilt is sometimes used to cover up other, less acceptable, feelings. You may feel guilty because you think your feelings are selfish, wrong, or different from what is expected.

You find well-wishers all around you cheering for your mate's recovery. What kind of a person would risk sabotaging the patient's progress by expressing worry or fear? What sort of individual feels sad and depressed when everyone else is being cheerful and optimistic?

Guilt comes when you realize you've done something hurtful to another person and feel disappointed in yourself. Many cardiac spouses feel responsible for their mate's heart disease or heart attacks. Louise, an assertive and outspoken woman, suffered guilt for many months because she and Jay had been arguing when his chest pain began. As she waited and watched in the hospital, she became convinced that if she hadn't raised her voice, hadn't felt so righteous about expressing her opinion, her darling Jay would not be in cardiac care. Even the lectures she attended at the hospital that helped define risk factors and methods of prevention did nothing to free Louise from her belief that she had caused Jay's heart attack. She couldn't look at the scar on Jay's chest, because it was such a powerful reminder of her fault.

Louise's case may seem extreme, but consider all the ways you feel responsible. You may feel guilty for using so much salt in your cooking over the last forty years. One man felt guilty because he agreed to drive his wife to the hospital rather than call 911. He believed that the damage to his wife's heart was increased because he lost precious minutes en route. Many spouses feel guilty because they didn't try to intervene in their mate's hospital care. Others feel especially guilty when they feel good (healthy), knowing their mates have heart disease; they may even try to hide how well they feel so their spouses won't feel envious.[5] Still others suffer because they initiate intervention and are unsuccessful. This was dramatized in the television movie "Heartsounds" (adapted from Martha Weinman Lear's book of the same title), when a cardiac spouse confronted the night nurse to persuade her to awaken the intern to change orders. The nurse refused because she was afraid she'd lose her job.

Although you probably know that you did the best you could in those circumstances, or realize that blaming yourself is unreasonable, it doesn't make guilt automatically disappear. Guilt becomes a problem when we don't understand it. If you feel guilty about your feelings, focus on them. Find out where your anger is coming from. Understand how you have been hurt. Examine your sadness and disappointment and experience those feelings fully.

If you feel guilty about hurting your spouse, assess your realistic responsibility.[6] Be accountable for your actions; apologize and make appropriate amends if the situation permits. Remember, your spouse's physical heart has healed. Your thoughts and feelings will not damage it.

A FEW POINTS TO REMEMBER ABOUT FEELINGS

- Feelings exist. You are not responsible for how you feel.
- It is normal to experience anger, fear, sadness, and guilt in response to the cardiac crisis.
- Depression is a normal response to a cardiac event, for patients, spouses, and other family members.
- Recognizing and identifying your feelings relieves and empowers you.
- Feelings provide an important source of information about yourself and your reactions to the world around you.
- Feelings change over time.
- Accepting and understanding your feelings gives you options about how and when to express them.
- Your feelings make you human, unique, and individual.
- Feelings connect you to other human beings.

Working with Changing Feelings

In a crisis, it is easy to be overwhelmed by your emotions. It may be difficult to sort out your feelings, much less do anything about them. This exercise will help you understand and cope with your feelings:

Step 1: First, you must recognize *what* you are feeling. By labeling your feelings, one by one, you can begin to clarify them.

Step 2: The next step is figuring out what you need. What would help to reduce your feelings of anger, fear, and sadness?

Step 3: The third and most crucial step involves

coming up with solutions. How can you help yourself? Once you know what you need, *you can take action.* Creative solutions require imagination and a positive attitude.

One way to keep yourself on track with this exercise is to put it all down in writing. I suggest you use a Heartmates® Feelings and Needs Assessment Diary[7] daily or at least regularly for a period of weeks. As your feelings and needs change over a period of time, you may find a weekly, and then monthly, evaluation sufficient. The pages of your diary may follow the form I suggest here:

HEARTMATES® FEELINGS AND NEEDS ASSESSMENT DIARY

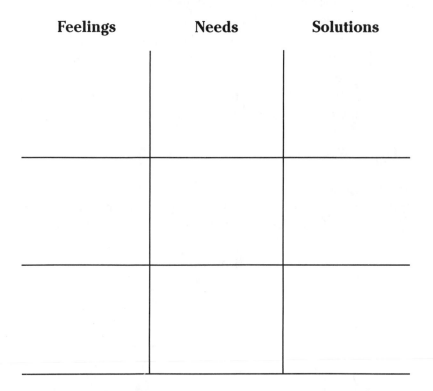

Feelings	Needs	Solutions

Under Feelings, write down a feeling you are having that is bothering you. (Begin the sentence with "I feel. . . .")

Under Needs, write down a need you have that is related to that feeling. (Begin the sentence with "I need. . . . ")

Under Solutions, write down as many actions as you can think of that can satisfy your need. (Begin each sentence with "I could. . . . ")

Here are some sample entries:

- I *feel* scared about money . . . I *need* information about our health benefits . . . I *could* call our accountant; I *could* call the social security office; I *could* look at our budget and financial records from last year; I *could* ask my husband to discuss our financial situation with me.
- I *feel* irritable about everything . . . I *need* some time for myself . . . I *could* take a nap; I *could* stay out of the kitchen and go to a restaurant for dinner tonight; I *could* weed my garden; I *could* sit down and read my favorite magazine; I *could* take a warm bubble bath; I *could* go for a long walk in the park.
- I *feel* afraid of being alone . . . I *need* to belong . . . I *could* call one of our kids to arrange a visit ; I *could* take a walk with my spouse; I *could* go to lunch with my best friend; I *could* reach out to talk to my next door neighbor; I *could* arrange to do some volunteer work with others through my church or community center.
- I *feel* sad . . . I *need* to allow and express my feelings . . . I *could* have a good cry; I *could* write a sad poem; I *could* ask my mate to hold me in his arms; I *could* share my sadness with a dear friend.

The Heartmates® Feelings and Needs Assessment Diary doesn't include space for the last step in the process. This is to *choose* one of your solutions and do it. Do whatever is necessary to make your solution a reality; it's always the final step in the process.

Very often the last step involves asking for what you want from other people. For most of us, this is the hardest part. But if you are willing to reach out - to your mate, to other family members, to friends - you will have a better chance of having your need for human support met.

Seeking Support

Working your way through a crisis is a highly personal experience. How many times have you sat up late at night worrying about your mate's health and wondering about your future? You may have thought that no one understands what you're going through. You're right. It's impossible for anyone to completely comprehend your experience. But that doesn't mean that no one cares.

There are times when solitude is exactly what you need. The soul-searching done when you are alone can be peaceful and healing. But you also need support. When you are hurting, it is especially important to allow yourself to be cared for. Each of us finds comfort in different ways. Express your fear and frustration to someone who is willing to listen patiently without making judgments. The kind word or warm hug you receive in return can be a much-needed gift of support. Or you may take solace from simply being in the company of a close friend.

Your friends and family may or may not be as supportive as you'd like. Even those who try their best may fail to offer their support in the right way.

David, a most pious man, climbed onto his roof during a flood. A boat going up the river stopped to invite him aboard. David refused, thanking them, because he believed the Lord would provide. He continued to sit on the roof and the water rose above the windows of his home. Another boat came by carrying people to dry land upstream, and they shouted up to him that they had room for him. Again David declined citing his belief that God would save him. The water rose up to the shingles of his roof. A helicopter flew by, saw David, and offered him a ladder to climb aboard. He responded, "Take your people to safety; I am not afraid, the Lord will provide." By dusk all but the peak of his roof was covered and the water was lapping at David's feet, and he cried, "Lord, why have you forsaken me?" There was a deafening thunder clap and a voice from the sky declared, "I didn't forsake you, David. Who do you think sent you two boats and a helicopter ?"

There is support available to you, but you need to follow some simple guidelines. You have to ask for what you need. Stay flexible. Support may not come packaged as you expect it. Reassess what you are getting from others. It may be exactly what you need, but not what you wanted. You need to do your part. Those who sit passively waiting usually miss the boat!

Despite their good intentions, others may unwittingly contribute to your sense of isolation. Early in the crisis, friends and family are apt to check in often. Their first question is about your partner's health. And rightly so. They express relief that he's doing well and recovering quickly. Most conversations end with the statement, "You must be thrilled that everything is going so well." Their concern is appreciated, but it's hardly an invitation to express your needs.

It's not so easy to ask a friend or relative for support, especially when they don't offer it directly. If your relationship is not characterized by sharing and intimacy, you may feel uncomfortable exposing your vulnerability and asking for help. But try your best to realize that this is an extraordinary situation. The normal rules of etiquette don't apply. Your friends and family may be unsure of the appropriate way to approach you. Perhaps they too present a cheerful face in order to keep up your spirits - and their own.

If you feel uneasy expressing your feelings, experiment a little, test the waters. Share one personal thing the next time a friend, relative, or neighbor calls. Once the initial barrier is broken, it will be easier to do so again. Or make it a habit to share something once each day. Assess how it goes. Don't overdo it; take small steps.

Accepting offers of meals or even financial aid from relatives is another way of letting them be there for you. Asking a friend to stop over for an hour so that you can take a break is not an imposition in a time of crisis. If you take the risk and ask for support, you may be pleasantly surprised by how eagerly it's given. And someday you may have the opportunity to return the favor.

Reaching Out

The best kind of support is reaching out to someone who is going through a similar experience. Other cardiac spouses are uniquely capable of relating to your feelings.

On the day of Marsh's surgery, I shared the waiting room with another cardiac spouse and her family. As the minutes crawled by, we each sat silently, alone with our thoughts. Finally, the door opened. The chaplain walked over and stood in front of me . Placing his hand on my shoulder, he said, "Your husband has come through fine; the surgery is over." My eyes filled with tears of relief. And through my tears, I saw that the other cardiac spouse was weeping, too.

During that seemingly unending block of time, we shared an intimacy that I'll never forget. The experience of the strong bond that developed so quickly between us forcefully reminded me that I was not alone. Later we kept each other company outside Intensive Care and visited each other's husbands in the post-surgical unit. Once we left the hospital we went our separate ways. But, in a very special way, we will always be connected.

One way to meet other cardiac spouses is to attend educational programs sponsored by your local hospital or clinic. In addition, your community may offer mental health programs that specialize in treating people affected by disease or trauma. Professional counseling during a time of crisis can be an important means of support. Contact with professionals who are sensitive to your needs may help you to cope with your loneliness and confusion.[8]

Ultimately, *you are not alone.* Reaching out for support is an absolutely essential step in recovery and in the process of reclaiming your health—and your life.

CHAPTER NOTES

1. For further understanding about the loneliness of the heartmate, see appendix D in this book.
2. See Stephanie Ericsson's *Companion Through The Darkness: Inner Dialogues on Grief,* (New York: Harper-Collins, 1993), for an eloquent and elegant experience of grieving. She describes the utility of anger on page 73.

3. Lesley Hazelton, *The Right to Feel Bad* (New York: Ballantine Books, 1984), pp. 196-197.
4. Henry David Thoreau, *Walden* (New York: Modern Library, 1950), p. 290.
5. The importance of the well spouse maintaining her health and her own separate life is discussed in an empowering way by Maggie Strong in her 1988 book, *Mainstay: For The Well Spouse of the Chronically Ill.*
6. It is useful to differentiate between needless guilt and guilt that is healthy and appropriate. See Judith Viorst, "Good as Guilt," chapter 9 in her book, *Necessary Losses* (New York: Fawcett Gold Medal, 1986), pp. 150-151, for a discussion of the healing value of making reparations for the wrongful act done.
7. Heartmates® Feelings and Needs Assessment Diary is adapted from Ellen Sue Stern, *Expecting Change* (New York: Poseidon Press, 1986), pp. 114-115.
8. Being alone is basic to the process of grief that all heartmates encounter, but that must be differentiated from loneliness. When the heartmate reaches out to tell someone her story and asks for support, she breaks through loneliness and achieves connection. Being vulnerable and sharing deep experience with another human being is a building block of establishing community. See appendix D of this book for a deeper look at loneliness and its antidote.

4

Keeping Your Head On Straight

The cardiac crisis plays havoc with your mind. From the very first instant, everything feels as though it's happening in double time. In a state of shock, you try desperately to clear your head and make the right moves. Inundated with information and advice, you struggle to make sense of it all.

A crisis affects the workings of your mind every bit as much as your feelings. As you try to comprehend what's happened, you may be surprised by your inability to think straight. It is common for cardiac spouses to have trouble concentrating and staying focused. Your ability to retain and comprehend information is affected, and you may feel as if you just can't track, are tuned out, or your thoughts are crazy or out of control.

In the first days after Marsh's heart attack, my mind seemed to have a life of its own. Over and over I was plagued by a litany of unanswerable questions. Instead

of thinking, "Well, I can see I'm in an awful situation, I need to figure out what to do, " I was fixated on the same material, my mind like a race car careening wildly around a speedway.
The logical questions I wish I could have asked were: "What is the priority here? What do I need to think about? What do I need to ask? What do I need to plan? What do I need to do?"

In any crisis it's hard to think, but you face an additional pressure: the difficult task of making immediate life-or-death decisions alone. Cardiac spouses, who are used to sharing decision making, now must do so without the input and support of their mates. There are pressing medical decisions to be made. At the onset of the crisis, when your mind is least functional, you are forced to act quickly and decisively.

Just hours after her husband's bypass surgery, as she was about to leave for home to get some much-needed rest, Helene was approached by her husband's medical team. They requested her permission to take Dennis back into surgery because of some unexpected internal bleeding. Overwhelmed by a sense of responsibility for his life, Helene could barely think, much less make one more decision. Through her blur of exhaustion, she summoned what was left of her energy and signed the papers.

We are generally advised to avoid decision making during a crisis. *Except for urgent problems that require immediate attention, cardiac spouses should put off decisions.* Premature decisions can be costly. Any change or decision that can be avoided in a crisis situation will reduce the stress and shock that the cardiac spouse, patient, and family are already suffering.

After Carole's fifty-four-year-old husband, Bill, suffered a cardiac arrest and a stroke, he was advised that he would need to spend the rest of his life in a nursing home. Carole was horrified at the idea but too distraught to protest. Like a zombie, she filled out the admittance forms. Bill was transferred from the hospital to the nursing home. Ten days later, he was literally climbing over the sides of his bed to use the bathroom. By this time, Carole had her wits about her. She and Bill decided that he should move back home and arrange for the assistance of a home health nurse, attend intensive physical therapy sessions, and participate in a cardiac rehabilitation program.

Directing Communications

No matter how you try to prevent it, you will, out of necessity, become the clearinghouse for news of your spouse's condition. It is a task that requires a clear head. Everyone - his parents, your children, your parents, friends, his boss and coworkers - must be informed. You need to analyze very carefully what to tell whom and when. There just isn't any way to soften bad news. Some cases are pretty straightforward; others are more sensitive.

My most delicate call was to Marsh's mother. Who would be more worried than his mother? Widowed twenty years ago when her husband died after a heart attack, she too has heart disease. I was afraid that the shock might aggravate her condition.

I had to be careful about when to call (certainly not at midnight when he was diagnosed). Luckily, Marsh's condition was not so critical that I couldn't wait for morning. Then, there was the question of how much to say. At that point I hadn't been given any test results or a prognosis. I wanted to give her an accurate picture without alarm-

ing her unnecessarily.

Comprehending the seriousness of the situation is another extremely difficult and draining task. Family members in other parts of the country may ask you to decide whether they should "be there." The complexities of family relationships make this a touchy issue. Your spouse may want to see some relatives, but not others. You are the designated spokesperson in the unenviable, uncomfortable position of having to say yes or no. You must be tactful, yet continue to respect your spouse's needs.

If your children are grown and away, you will want to consider seriously and carefully whether *you* want them to come home. You are entitled to express your preference. They have the right to decide what they will do. You need to weigh the emotional benefits of their presence against the potential disruption in all of your lives. How can you keep yourself from feeling as if you have to take care of them too? Will you be loving and supportive to each other, or will old family conflicts flare up and cause additional pain?

One man thought twice before calling their son, away at college during exam week, to inform him that his mother had suffered a heart attack. Another cardiac spouse made the decision, with her fingers crossed, not to send for their two daughters, who were off at music camp. Still another knew instinctively that their thirty-year-old daughter wouldn't rest easy until she saw her father with her own two eyes.

Some patients are adamant about not wanting anyone but you at the hospital. Some parents don't want to "bother the children," or have them "see Dad this way." They would prefer the kids to come when they're out of the hospital and feeling less vulnerable at home. Others are comforted by having the whole family gathered around.

Director of Communications is the position you assume, as you manage the information clearinghouse. Your access to the patient makes you the obvious source of information for family and friends. Because you are closest to the situation, you are expected to relay messages and provide medical reports. Everyone means well and sends love and best wishes. Their support is appreciated, but it's exhausting to repeat every detail of recovery each time someone calls. You wish you had a press secretary so the information could be passed more efficiently.

How can you think about everyone else's needs when you can barely get your own head on straight? You may be asked indirectly whether you think your mate will survive. You may not be prepared or willing to confront this question. Young children may ask directly, "Is my Daddy going to die?" Is there a way to provide an honest and realistic answer and still manage to comfort your child? What is good counsel for your grown son, who is trying to make a decision about leaving his own family in another part of the country to be with his parents?

You cannot always make wise decisions when you are dealing with the unknown. What if your mate doesn't survive? Would it be better or worse if the children were present? What are the psychological risks if they aren't there and their parent dies? There are no easy answers. Good judgment is difficult when your mind is scattered and you are confused.

Don't let other people's urgency and fear pressure you. You may be too upset or exhausted to make any decisions except for those that are absolutely critical. And remember that "I don't know" is a perfectly acceptable answer. *You're not responsible for knowing everything.* You can't predict the future.

What You Need to Know about Your Thinking

It usually takes time, sometimes as much as several months, for your mind to return to its normal level of functioning. Some cardiac spouses have chronic problems concentrating and remembering details, since they are still so preoccupied. One woman who was habitually a voracious reader, couldn't focus her attention long enough to follow magazine recipes for the first six months after her mate's heart attack. Another spouse had to bring work home with him, because his shortened attention span caused him to fall behind on the job.

I was particularly unnerved by an incident that showed how distracted I was. One day, several weeks after Marsh's heart attack, I was driving home from work. When I turned off the ignition, I was surprised to find myself in the driveway of our old house. We hadn't lived there for over two years. I must have been driving on automatic pilot, or maybe I unconsciously wanted to turn time back. In either case, I felt scared by how disoriented I was. I wondered if it was safe for me to drive. I even thought I might be going crazy.

Uncontrollable circular thinking is another symptom that affects cardiac spouses. Like a broken record, your mind goes over and over the events of your spouse's cardiac event. You may repeat the same stories, lose your train of thought, or be totally unable to think about anything else. You may find this repetitive thinking occurring for many weeks into the recovery period.

Another phenomenon that is instinctively triggered when people confront sudden and unexpected loss is a mechanism called *life review*.[1] The most important events of your life are quickly and vividly recalled, as they are when you have a near miss while driving on the highway and your whole life flashes by you before you've braked to a complete halt. If you recall getting the news of your spouse's heart attack, you may remember experiencing a partial life review. In less than a minute you mentally saw the highlights of your whole marriage. While this was happening, you may have momentarily lost track of time or been thoroughly absorbed in another world. None of this means that you've lost your mind. On the contrary, life review is a natural process which prepares you to deal with loss.

It is normal and healthy to relive your experience. Your mind is trying to make sense of shocking and chaotic events. The process of mental repetition brings order out of chaos. Repeating the details of your experience aloud, you clarify and deepen your understanding.

While the urgent need to share your experience diminishes over time, cardiac spouses exchange stories for years with as much intensity as if the events had just happened. Although many years have passed, I still get emotional while thinking and talking about Marsh's heart attacks. Be kind and patient with yourself. Be sure to give yourself as much time as you need. Meeting with other cardiac spouses will give you the opportunity to tell your story long after friends and neighbors have lost interest. Sharing serves a purpose; perhaps it is even necessary if you are to integrate your experience, recover from the cardiac crisis, and continue your personal growth.

Surviving the acute crisis doesn't automatically relieve the stresses and pressures that you know exist. A number of detailed responsibilities follow you home from the hospital. You must be attentive and alert to communicate with the doctor, supervise your mate's medications, and structure a new dietary plan. Beyond coping with daily tasks, you need your mind clear to make ongoing decisions and to confront the deeper meaning of the crisis.

Untangling the Web

Your thoughts and your feelings are closely intertwined. Anxiety makes your thinking less rational. And when you're not thinking rationally, your anxiety accelerates - a vicious cycle. In a crisis, powerful feelings wrap themselves around your mind like a blanket, suffocating you. No matter how hard you try to concentrate, you end up panicky and confused. Fears about the future paralyze you until you can't think. Even after you make a decision, your fear can stop you, freezing any action.

If you're blaming yourself for not being more organized and decisive, *stop*. It's very likely that your feelings are getting in the way. Whether you are seeking information, have an important decision to make, or need the solutions to more unanswered questions, the first step is to deal with your feelings. Acknowledging your feelings is important. If you know what you're feeling, you can calm down and begin to think logically.

Gathering information is a positive way to dispel anxiety. Most people cope better when they have the whole story. Without it, your imagination runs wild, creating scenarios far worse than reality. If you're like most cardiac spouses, you probably have a slew of unspoken, unaddressed, and unanswered questions. They may torment you when you are trying to sleep or pop up at odd times, catching you unaware. You may find them circling around and around in your head without any landing gear. First, organize your questions into a list. I strongly recommend keeping a pad of paper and a pencil handy, day and night. Write down any question that comes up. Or, you can ask your questions aloud to yourself or to someone willing to listen.

Once you have access to your questions, you can categorize them. Separate them into two groups: those that are unanswerable and those that have potential answers. For the time being, set aside the questions that don't have answers. Focus on questions to which there *are* answers in order to reduce your anxiety and empower yourself toward action. Using your mind will reassure you that you haven't lost it.

Next, divide your questions into two subgroups: informational questions and decision-making questions. Informational questions provide data about your mate's condition, prognosis, and the repercussions of heart disease. With this information you will begin to see the truths of your situation. Some sample informational questions include:

- What causes heart disease?
- What are the newest medical treatments that may pro long my spouse's life?
- How long will recovery take?
- What life-style limitations can we anticipate?
- When is it safe to resume sexual activity?

Obtaining information is an ongoing process. A trip to the library to borrow material about heart disease will provide you with some valuable information. So can attendance at lectures and participation in seminars for cardiac patients and their families. Not only will you get answers to your questions, but you may learn something that can directly improve your spouse's recovery. If you aren't accustomed to being persistent and assertive, you may find seeking information difficult but empowering.

You may find yourself hesitant to ask strangers about highly personal things, but try not to let fear or embarrassment stop you from finding out what you need to know. Sources for information include:

American Heart Association National Center
7320 Greenville Avenue
Dallas, Texas 75231
(Use your phone book to locate your state office)

American Association of Cardiovascular and Pulmonary Rehabilitation (AACVPR)
7611 Elmwood Avenue, Suite 201
Middleton, Wisconsin 53562
(608) 831-6989

Heartmates®
P.O. Box 16202
Minneapolis, Minnesota 55416
(612) 929-3331; fax (612) 929-6395
e-mail address: heartmates@aol.com
WorldWideWeb url: http://www.heartmates.com/

Well Spouse Foundation (a national network of well spouses of the chronically ill)
P.O. Box 801
New York City, New York 10023

Harvard Heart Letter (monthly newsletter from Harvard Medical School)
P.O. Box 420234
Palm Coast, Florida 32142-0234
(800) 829-9171

Cardiac rehabilitation programs at your local hospital, YMCA, or Jewish Community Center

Write to, call, or visit any of these organizations. What you learn may benefit you and your mate directly. Seeking, getting, and understanding information on heart disease and recovery can help you focus your thinking, strengthen your foundation for decision- making, reduce your feelings of helplessness, and increase your sense of control.

Mustering up courage to discuss sexual activity with your physician might turn out to be well worth your while. Steady your mind and seek answers to your questions. It will only increase your confidence in yourself as you cope with your crisis.

Decision-making questions have a different purpose from informational questions. They are geared to help you think about issues so you can make informed decisions. Some sample decision-making questions include:

- How should I inform family members about a change in my spouse's condition?
- Should my spouse go ahead with bypass surgery?
- Should we plan a winter vacation in the sun?
- What financial adaptations do we need to make?
- What changes need I consider about my career or retirement?
- What life-style changes should we make? Should I make?

Accentuate the Positive

Often cardiac spouses feel depressed and pessimistic even after the doctor indicates that a high quality of life is the most likely recovery for the patient. But you don't have to stay stuck with your negative reactions. You can learn thinking skills that will enhance your recovery from the cardiac crisis.

Dr. Martin E. P. Seligman, who has studied help-lessness and pessimism juxtaposed to empowerment and optimism, explains, "When we encounter adversity, we react by thinking about it. Our thoughts rapidly congeal into beliefs....Usually the negative beliefs that follow adversity are inaccurate....These beliefs may become so habitual we don't even realize we have them unless we stop and focus on them. And they don't just sit there idly; they have consequences. The beliefs are the direct causes of what we feel and what we do next."[2]

The goal of learning to think positively is to increase your control over how you perceive your present situation and see more clearly how you can positively affect your future. The first step to achieve control and act more positively is to recognize when you are caught in a pessimistic thinking style. Once you recognize your negative thoughts, you can do something positive about them. You may not be experienced at analyzing your thinking patterns, but you can learn! That is the key to gaining control. Go over these four steps designed to help you examine your thoughts.

1. **Evidence** is about accuracy and facts. Verify the accuracy of what you tell yourself. This technique involves asking yourself the question: What is the evidence for my belief? Searching for evidence that points out the distortions in your catastrophic beliefs is the first step. Look for evidence that shifts the focus away from blaming yourself or your spouse for your cardiac situation.

You tell yourself and believe that your healthy food plan is "shot" and another cardiac event is imminent.

Why? Because your spouse ate chocolate cake and ice cream at your grandson's birthday party. Look at all the evidence. Count the actual fat grams and calories your mate consumed at the party. Reread results of his latest cholesterol tests, and acknowledge weight loss by noting what the bathroom scale reads. Put the alleged crime in perspective.

2. **Alternatives** is about looking for the multiple causes for what has happened, and not just focusing on the most pessimistic. Scan your understanding for all possible contributing causes, and focus on the change-able, the specific, and the nonpersonal causes. Your task is to look for and generate alternative causes, rather than succomb to the old habit of latching onto the most nega-tive cause.

Remind yourself that maintaining total deprivation of favorite foods is impossible for long periods of time. This understanding can ease your dis-ease when your mate eats cake and ice cream on your grandson's birth-day. Taking a break from your regular diet on a special occasion can be thought of as a celebration, not a failure; a celebration of both your grandson's birthday and of your spouse's recovery. Experience your gratitude that your mate is here, alive and recovering, to share the birthday celebration. And after a break, you both can return to your heart-healthy food plan with renewed commitment.

3. **Implications** is about the likelihood of a nega-tive result in the event that the negative belief is correct. The question to ask is: Even if my belief *is* correct, what does that really imply?

When you look at the evidence, you may find it true that eating chocolate cake and ice cream at the birth-day party means that your mate exceeded his daily fat gram goal and he may even have temporarily gained a pound or two. The facts don't necessarily imply that he is suicidal, lacks will power, or that he should give up the food plan permanently because he failed on one occasion. The real implication may only be that your spouse is human!

4. **Usefulness** is about judging the consequences of holding a particular belief, even if it is true. The question to ask yourself is: Is the belief destructive? Even if the belief is true now, is the situation changeable? And if it is changeable, how can you go about changing it? Dwelling on the negative belief won't resolve anything. By focusing on what you can do, looking for solutions, you are more likely to achieve a sense of progress, of moving on with your life.

Right now your spouse may lack the necessary will power to succeed with the heart-healthy food plan. Rather than let go of the plan, focus on methods he can use to strengthen his will.

Betty and Dan illustrate the importance of learning to think positively. Betty came home unexpectedly and found Dan smoking in the garage. In a flash, her thoughts jumped to her most catastrophic explanation for his smoking. He didn't love her! He would rather smoke cigarettes and die than live to grow old with her. She accused him of total irresponsibility; she called him names, and stalked out of the garage. Betty was determined never to discuss what had happened with Dan. She was furious and felt deeply hurt.

The incident might have ended in a stalemate, with Betty alienated from Dan and no resolution in sight. Using her new thinking techniques Betty came to see things differently. It *was* irresponsible for Dan to be smoking because of his cardiac condition and rehabilitation program, but *total irresponsibility* was a catastrophic exaggeration. Dan has managed his food plan reasonably well, and is devout about his cardiovascular exercise. It *was* serious that Dan lied about having quit smoking, but assuming that everything Dan says is a lie keeps Betty feeling hurt and hopeless.[3] Using her optimistic thinking tools, Betty recognized her feelings and decided to discuss the situation with Dan. Communication opened between them, and together they laid the groundwork for further discussion as well as support for Dan to continue his difficult struggle to quit smoking.

Five Elements of Clear Thinking Before Making a Decision

Crisis is not an ideal time to make decisions. You feel especially vulnerable, unable to think clearly. And yet you are expected to make important decisions that just can't be postponed. It helps to approach the process in an organized fashion. I have reduced the process into five components to make it simpler and less overwhelming. Consider each of these elements before you make a decision.

1. **Priority.** How important is the decision?
2. **Involving Others.** Is this a decision to be made alone or with others?
3. **Time.** How urgent is the decision?
4. **Action**. Is this an active or receptive decision?
5. **Purpose**. What is my purpose and goal?

1. WHAT'S THE PRIORITY

It is vital that you differentiate between big and

little decisions. Your energy is limited, and you are more likely to spin your wheels unless you clarify the priorities. Once you decide that something is really significant, you can concentrate your attention and make a decision based on your assessment of all the possible consequences. If it's truly important, it deserves your most mindful consideration. If it's not a high priority, you can let it wait.

Of course, when you are upset, fatigued, and confused, it isn't always obvious which decisions are critical or urgent. What you really need is perspective. Ask a trusted friend to look at your list of decisions; it might help you to see more clearly. I advise asking yourself questions that will help you assess and clarify the priority of an issue. Ask yourself how important the issue is to you, your spouse, your family? Will it have a long-term effect on your future or is it something that will soon be forgotten? How much does it concern you? If making a medical decision is consistently on your mind, take care of it before moving on to other things. If life-style issues are most confusing, give them your attention.

You also need to verify that your concerns are realistic. Sharing your list with someone who is compassionate but less involved can give you the opportunity to look at the issue in light of the bigger picture. Once you have arranged your decisions in order of priority, based on the intensity of your concern, long-range consequences, and a reality check, you can deal with them one at a time.

2. INVOLVING OTHERS

The next consideration is how to make a decision. Since you are the healthy one, it stands to reason that you should make the decisions. On the other hand, they directly affect your mate. Certain decisions may seem too trivial, a waste of his energy, and others so stressful as to place him at risk. Some cardiac spouses assume full responsibility, choosing to exclude their spouses, other family members, medical staff, or trusted friends who can offer suggestions and provide another perspective.

This can be controlling and isolating. Remember, results of decisions often have an impact on the whole cardiac family. In the best circumstances, you hope you are able to take other people's needs into consideration.

Making decisions alone or cooperatively is a matter of individual style. In a crisis people usually fall back on what is most familiar, but that may not be the best prescription for the situation at hand. If you are a person who usually thinks and decides alone, you may want to consider the advantages of asking others for their input. And if you are a person who tends to rely on others, you might consider thinking these decisions through on your own. Whichever style works best for you, your goal is to make the best decision possible for all involved.

3. THE ASPECT OF TIME

Timing is yet another serious element in decision making. There are decisions that need to be made instantaneously, and there is plenty of time to plan others. Maintaining clarity can be tricky. In a crisis, your sense of time becomes distorted. Time can seem to stretch out to infinity when you're waiting to hear how your spouse has come through a surgical procedure. Or a long time can pass in the flash of a millisecond when you picture your years together before the cardiac crisis. When you are making a decision, it is important to differentiate urgency or the need for speed from adequate time to make the wisest decision.

Barely two months after Marsh's recovery from a second mild heart attack, his cardiologist suggested that he have an angiogram. His opinion afterward: no surgery indicated; proceed with conservative treatment, including diet, exercise, and medication.
Thoroughly frightened by two heart attacks, we decided to seek a second opinion.
A second cardiologist advised the exact opposite, saying, "If I were you, I'd have surgery as soon as possible." We were stunned! It never dawned on us that getting a second opinion would complicate our decision. We naively had expected it to verify that Marsh's cardiologist was "right" and to reassure us because we felt so vulnerable and powerless.
We had been hoping to increase our security. Instead, our anxiety was multiplied.
Our purpose was clear. We were committed to doing whatever would be best for Marsh's health. But what was best? We struggled with the decision for a week, going over the advantages and disadvantages in our minds.
We felt powerfully drawn toward a decision in favor of surgery. We both wanted Marsh to live the active life of a normal forty-five year old. If we chose surgery, we thought our panic would diminish, and that somehow Marsh would be safer. And it would feel as if we were doing something - anything - to relieve the mounting tension.
But the disadvantages were obvious, too. Having gone through two recent recovery periods, surgery would mean starting over a third time. It would take another three to six months for Marsh to rebuild his physical strength and endurance. We knew that bypass surgery was no guarantee that Marsh would avoid a third heart attack or that he would live a longer life.
Marsh's cardiologist gave us articles to read from the highly respected "New England Journal of Medicine" that corroborated his interpretation. He reminded us that time was in our favor; cardiac research was rapidly developing new technology that was less dangerous and more

effective. Since heart disease was progressive, it would be wise to save surgery, an invasive, risky treatment, until it was necessary. He assured us that if anything in Marsh's condition changed, surgery would be seriously considered. From beginning to end, our cardiologist was logical, informative, and respectful of every question we asked.

Finally, we decided. Marsh would go with the more conservative treatment; he would not have bypass surgery. Just reaching a decision helped to reduce our anxiety and stress. Eventually, Marsh stopped feeling like a time bomb about to explode. Because we had shared the decision-making process, we both felt unequivocally committed to Marsh's recovery plan. He reaffirmed his choice with his strong commitment to regular exercise in a cardiac rehabilitation class. He took his medications regularly, and he assumed responsibility for moderating his diet.

Almost two years passed before circumstances changed radically. One morning Marsh awakened with severe chest pains that were only sporadically relieved by nitroglycerin. Walking the half block from the parking lot to his office left him short of breath. Urgency and fear returned to our lives. Our cardiologist scheduled an angiogram and surgery for the following day. Now our decision was urgent: Marsh's life was on the line. And again we were faced with a choice. This time the choice was to have bypass surgery. Although we were scared about the surgery and disappointed that it was necessary after all the changes Marsh had made, we were satisfied that it was the right choice.

4. ACTION AND INACTION

Most people consider decision making as exclusively active. We think that making a decision means taking a stand or doing something. In fact, decision making often involves acceptance and trust, and being receptive to someone else's judgment. Accepting the fact that there is nothing to be done, is actually doing something. A decision not to act, not to schedule bypass surgery after Marsh's heart attacks, was as much of a decision as choosing to do so two years later.

Every decision you make is simultaneously saying "yes" to something, and "no" to something else. Every "yes" is also "no"! We generally ignore what needs a "no," because it may be uncomfortable or unpleasant. Your decision to establish a heart-healthy diet requires you to say "no" to fatty meats and salty soups.

Whether your decision requires action or maintenance of the status quo, try to be positively involved in the process. This means initiating action when it is appropriate and choosing to remain still when that will be most beneficial. Accepting inaction in the face of danger requires courage and faith. There's little in life that is more demanding than simply waiting and being receptive to what comes.

5. ESTABLISHING GOALS

Finally, you'll need to explore your underlying purpose so you can define your goals - it's a prerequisite to good decision making. Goals guide our actions, and are positive in that they are future oriented and enhance hope and optimism. *Achieving goals, short or long range, is less important than having them.*

To establish purpose, you will have to ask the question, "Why?" Struggling with that "why?" may not yield a specific answer, but it will help you pinpoint and solidify your goals. Your purpose might be general, like expressing the love that you feel for your spouse, or specific, like understanding and supporting a new exercise regimen. Your purpose forms the natural foundation for the decisions you want to make.

Bernice, a talented and respected counselor, became a cardiac spouse just after her fiftieth birthday. About six months after her husband's heart attack, she asked me to help her with a career decision. Bernice and Bernard's financial situation was secure. He had a solid offer to sell his small business, and decided, at age fifty-three, to retire early.

Until Bernard's heart attack, their marriage had been satisfying, but secondary. With two full-time careers and no children, they were both accustomed to being independent and going their own ways. Bernard's illness brought them closer together. Bernice discovered that her husband meant more to her than she had ever thought. Confronted with the possibility of losing him, she realized that she wanted to make their relationship a higher priority in her life.

Bernice's goal was to reorganize her time so that it matched her new values. She tried to weigh the pros and cons of keeping or giving up her career. Retiring would mean that she and Bernard would have more time together. They would be able to relax, spend time quietly at the shore, and escape the stress of city life.

On the surface, it seemed like a perfect solution. Her family had never been supportive of her need for a career; it had always been a disappointment to them that Bernice hadn't chosen to be a homemaker and mother. On the other hand, her work was a big part of what made her feel valued. Having her own earned income, although it was much smaller than Bernard's, enhanced her feelings of independence and provided a sense of maturity that parenthood may otherwise have given her. And without her job, she felt as if she would be giving up the only thing that she could really call her own.

As she reexamined her priorities, Bernice realized how much she valued her marriage and her career. Both emerged as powerful rivals for top of her list of priorities, so she decided to choose a workable, meaningful compromise. She elected to compress her working days to Tuesdays, Wednesdays, and Thursdays, an arrangement that freed up the rest of her week to spend with Bernard. Staying in touch with her original goal helped Bernice turn an "either/or" decision into a "both/and" opportunity.

Staying in touch with your purpose while you act is difficult, particularly during the acute phase of the cardiac crisis, and even as you reorient your life during recovery. The cardiac crisis often opens for consideration old values you have taken for granted, but doesn't necessarily offer answers. Major decisions require investigation and understanding followed by realignment of your actions with your carefully considered values. Taking time to think about your decisions can keep you connected to the purpose behind your actions. And committing them to paper, as you write what you feel, can help you stay on track. Here is a Heartmates® Guide to use as you work through the process of decision making.

HEARTMATES® GUIDE FOR DECISION MAKING

1. What is the decision facing me? (State it as clearly as possible.)
2. What is my purpose for making this decision?
3. What options are open to me that would help me achieve my purpose? (List all options you can think of, including those you know you would not ultimately choose.)
4. What are the positives and negatives (the costs) of each of these options? What can I predict as the result or consequence of each option? To me? To my spouse? To our family? To others?

5. What feelings do I have as I consider this decision?
6. Are there things I need to know, to learn about, before I can think through this decision? How can I get the information I need?
7. Once you have considered these questions, make your decision, and commit it to writing: "I have decided to . . . " or "I choose to. . . ."
8. How do I feel about having made this decision? Is ambivalence or another feeling getting in the way of my acting on my choice?
9. Don't avoid necessary decisions. Not deciding is a decision.
10. Remember your original purpose as you act on your decision. Use this guide to keep you connected to your goals.
11. Celebrate your success!

Considering the Deeper Questions

The cardiac crisis brings you face to face with how much control you have. Sometimes, no matter how well informed or decisive you are, there are areas over which you have little or no authority. You can't make heart disease disappear. You can't change what has already happened to you and your mate because of heart disease. You can't even change how you feel about it. Your power is limited to choosing what your attitude will be about what is happening. You can be in charge of the way you will accept and adapt to a new reality, a new life.

Living with unanswerable questions is painful. It is a rare and unusual individual who would choose uncertainty over security. But accepting your powerlessness also has its rewards.

Your day-to-day life has been ruptured by a cardiac crisis. All your perceptions are altered. The result can be an awakening to a new level of thinking, deeper than your prevailing habit permits. You may experience it as a sense that something is different. You may have a momentary flash that "life is not forever" or that "this relationship is precious." Many cardiac spouses do not recognize these flashes, because the everyday mind is so insistent and demanding. Those who have this revelation describe it as a whisper rising in the rare moments when the mind calms down.

The whisper directs the cardiac spouse to the deeper questions that are an integral, though often buried, part of the cardiac crisis. These questions invite you to explore issues beyond medications, diets, and daily routines. They provoke serious thought about mortality, purpose, and the meaning of life. They ask you to look at yourself in relation to the larger world, to other cardiac spouses, to all people in pain, and even to all others on our planet.

The everyday part of the mind races clamorously, scrambling for concrete answers; it loves cholesterol levels and milligrams, the countable, the measurable, and the knowable. The whispering question doesn't seek the right answer; it only needs permission to be heard. Simply contemplating issues and struggling to understand questions will enable you to grow emotionally.

Sure, it's easier to stay involved with the practical questions; the unknown is so disconcerting. Many cardiac spouses may have conscientiously avoided such questions since childhood or adolescence. Others have outgrown the answers they accepted then, but haven't had the occasion to reexamine them until now. Still others may be disillusioned by the idealistic answers of youth. It is natural to push nagging questions away by saying, "None of this really matters," or, "I haven't got time to think about this, because I have to take care of the everyday tasks that fill my life," or, like Scarlett O'Hara, promise yourself to think about it tomorrow.

I propose that recovery is an ideal time to ponder the realm of meaning and purpose. The cardiac crisis has made you vulnerable, and you are more likely to see the gravity of those deeper questions about the meaning and quality of life. The protection of normal, daily life and the illusions of being powerful and in full control over your life have broken down, so in a time of crisis the whisper can be heard.

Should you choose to respond, make sure to give yourself some regular quiet time. Find a place where you can think undisturbed; go for a walk, take a long, hot bath, or sit in your favorite easy chair. Start a diary or a journal to keep an ongoing record of your experience for later reflection.[4] Or pursue your thoughts and questions by sharing them with a trusted friend or talking with a mentor or a spiritual guide. There is no "right" way to ponder the deeper questions. Whatever your individual style is, take advantage of the opportunity.

SOME THOUGHTS ON THINKING

- Limited concentration and inability to focus are normal responses to a cardiac crisis.
- Normal thinking patterns return more slowly than feelings.
- Reviewing the events of your cardiac story is a natural and healing mental response.
- Repetition transforms chaos and confusion into a sense of order and meaning.
- Recognizing feelings is a first step to untangling thoughts.
- Sharing thoughts can give you another's perspective

and a valuable reality check.
- Postpone unnecessary decision making whenever possible until you have control over your thinking.
- The everyday, rational part of your mind is an important resource in decision making.
- The quiet, abstract part of your mind connects you to questions of meaning and to your internal wisdom.

CHAPTER NOTES

1. Rhoda F. Levin, "Life Review: A Natural Process," in *Readings in Psychosynthesis: Theory, Process, and Practice* (Toronto, Canada: Ontario Institute for Studies in Education), pp. 82 - 96.
2. Martin E. P. Seligman, Ph.D. *Learned Optimism* (New York:Alfred A. Knopf, Inc., 1990), pp. 221 - 225. This important book presents a powerful argument and practical techniques for overcoming pessimistic thinking. Most of us believe mistakenly that if we can control our feelings, we will be less helpless.

   Personal control is the opposite of helplessness; it indicates the ability to think about, decide, and take personal action to change things.

   It has been shown statistically that the more changes (stressors) a person encounters in a period of time, the greater the risk to the immune system, for infectious illness, for depression, even heart attacks and cancer. (Loss, pessimism, depression, catecholamine depletion, endorphin secretion depletion, immuune suppression, disease, p.182.)

   The other major factor defining risk for illness and predicting recovery is "social support." The capacity to love and sustain meaningful friendships, as opposed to being friendless and isolated, can be a marker for recovery.

For those interested in the topic of changing negative thinking, I also recommend John Roger and Peter McWilliams book *You Can't Afford the Luxury of a Negative Thought* (Los Angeles: Prelude Press, 1988).

3. Mary Hayes-Grieco calls hope a discipline, not a feeling, in her book *The Kitchen Mystic: Spiritual Lessons Hidden in Everyday Life* (Center City, MN: Hazelden Books, 1992). "Hope is a set of behaviors and attitudes you adopt to carry you forward as if yourlife matters, even though at the moment you may feel that it doesn't. When you are facing a time of emotion and lack of direction, it is an act of hope to tend to health habits like eating and sleeping and to keep a minimum level of beauty and order in your appearance and environment."

4. Journal keeping can be an aid in clarifying thoughts as well as helping to process grief. A useful resource tool for journal keeping is Christina Baldwin's 1990 book, *Life's Companion: Journal Writing as a Spiritual Quest*, published by Bantam Books.

5

Shifting Responsibility

Before the cardiac crisis, you had a busy, active life. You probably weren't looking for any extra work or stress. Whether at home, in your marriage, or in your career, you could handle the daily demands of your life.

But from the moment your mate became a cardiac patient, your responsibilities changed. Regardless of what the division of labor had been prior to the cardiac event, you now find yourself saddled with both your mate's and your own shares.

In the acute stage of the crisis, your responsibilities simply snowballed. Suddenly, you were in charge of medical decisions, financial arrangements, and the emotional needs of your family. At the most extreme, your mate was bedridden, perhaps unable to speak. His only responsibility was to rest so that his heart would heal. You were responsible for everything else.

The dramatic switch in responsibility is intensified because *you are in crisis.* Your anxiety is heightened and even simple decisions seem overwhelming. Normal demands seem heavier and less manageable. And the crisis creates new jobs and still more responsibilities as you must inform family and friends, and run the household single-handedly.

Once your mate returns home, your hands are full in other ways. Because economic considerations make hospital stays shorter, you end up having to give your mate semi-skilled nursing care. Your spouse's physical activity is limited, and he still spends much of his time in bed. The majority of *your* time is spent preparing and serving meals, changing bedding, and monitoring medications.

Believing that homecoming will be a joyous celebration is overly simplistic. Most of us look forward to the end of hospitalization, but because of inexperience we can't anticipate the complexity of the situation. Spouses and family members are both struggling with their own understanding of the meaning of heart disease and hospitalization. Established patterns and daily routines have been disrupted and redefined. A new chain of command excluding the patient has developed within the family. You may feel discouraged or resentful about being questioned or second-guessed for decisions made during hospitalization. Family dynamics can never return to the idealized vision of how they were before heart disease; you can't change or erase what has happened, nor can you control other family members' reactions to the cardiac crisis.

Patients too have been deeply affected by hospitalization. Much of their energy is consumed consciously or unconsciously confronting the awesome issue of their own mortality. Heart disease doesn't happen just to "perfect" families; it happens in families that are resilient and strong as well as those for whom heart disease feels like the "last straw" in the midst of chaos. Earlier unresolved family issues, like alcoholism, abuse, or chronic unemployment, can heighten the stress of adjusting to heart disease. Some patients return home to find that their power in the household and their responsibility for discipline of children has been usurped by their well spouse. Others come home, feeling weak and unsure about their health and future, and feel the burden of an increased dependence on the part of spouse and children. Still others may find spouses and children have become so independent that patients feel replaced and unneeded.

As if your immediate family were not enough, you find it also incumbent on you to make sure that friends and relatives don't overstay their visits. You feel it's up to you to make sure that your mate doesn't get overly taxed or exhausted. And, despite your own fatigue, you may feel obliged to play hostess by taking reservations for visiting hours, serving coffee and sweets, and cleaning up after the guests are gone.

Entertaining only adds to your stress when you are coping with a crisis. Some visitors are a source of comfort, and you welcome them with open arms, but others are more of a hindrance than a help. Some guests stop by, pay attention to the patient, eat a bite, and disappear (sort of like doting grandparents who leave before the diapers have to be changed). Other visitors arrive with food, flowers, and gifts of love and support.

This is not the time for you to put other people's needs first. You have stretched yourself to your physical and emotional limits. Kudos of appreciation for you are in order. Assuming a cardiac spouse's responsibilities deserves respect and recognition from you, your mate, and others. And yet you may be tempted to tolerate inconvenient or insensitive visitors out of politeness. You may feel guilty turning away guests who might cheer up your mate. But this is your home, too. If you can, try to overcome your feelings of obligation. If you feel you have to stand on ceremony with some people, ask them to visit at a later date.

Once you enter the recovery phase, new and different responsibilities emerge. If your spouse has had to face early retirement, you may be financially pressured and have to become the sole breadwinner. Running back and forth between your job and home adds more anxiety and stress.

Cardiac patients are often depressed, and by default they leave the majority of daily responsibilities to you. Even if your mate is recovering relatively smoothly, you might still spend hours catering heart-healthy meals or running to the pharmacy. Or, perhaps months down the road, you find yourself stuck, unable to stop constantly "baby-sitting" your mate.

Shifting responsibility is one of the most complex issues you face. On the surface, the choice seems obvious: Your mate needs help, so it's natural for you to assume the responsibility. And the fact that he's depending on you makes you want to rise to the occasion.

Because of the unexpected and sudden onset of the cardiac crisis, you simply take on whatever needs to be done. You may believe that you have no choice and that loving your spouse means picking up all the slack.

How much responsibility you take on can be measured quite easily. Look at how you spend your time. However, understanding your patterns of responsibility, and how much you and your mate depend on each other, is more complicated. Patterns that take years to develop become firmly entrenched in your relationship. Caring for your sick spouse has either cemented existing patterns, or created entirely new ones.

You may or may not be aware of how your responsibilities have changed. Each new task that you have added to your repertoire may have been a conscious choice. Or you may have gradually added more and more without being aware of it. You feel as if all your existing responsibilities are equally important and you can't alter them. But before you can consider any future action, you need to be aware of how your responsibilities have already changed.

Answer the following questions to delineate your changing responsibilities. Begin by evaluating your "normal" (pre-cardiac crisis) responsibilities. Then, look at your new responsibilities.

HEARTMATES® RESPONSIBILITY QUESTIONNAIRE

Before the cardiac crisis:

1. Which spouse took more responsibility in each of the following areas:

_____ earning a living
_____ handling the family finances
_____ meals
_____ housework
_____ yard work
_____ parenting your children
_____ caring for aging parents
_____ social and recreational activities
_____ your relationship with each other
_____ spiritual life

2. In what ways was your spouse dependent on you?
3. In what ways were you dependent on your spouse?
4. Have the two of you become more or less dependent on each other throughout the life of your relationship?

5. Did you consider yourself:

_____ independent
_____ too independent
_____ dependent
_____ too dependent
_____ interdependent
_____ responsible
_____ overresponsible
_____ underresponsible

Since the cardiac crisis:

1. What responsibilities are different now? What do you do now that's different? How do you feel about your new responsibilities?
2. List ways in which you are more dependent on your spouse now.
3. List ways in which you are less dependent on your spouse now.
4. In what ways is your spouse more dependent on you now?
5. In what ways is your spouse more independent from you now?

Identifying and understanding changes in responsibility earmark the beginning of your recovery. Whether you have taken on more responsibility consciously or as a matter of course, these new patterns form the foundation of your relationship. Habits establish themselves quickly. Temporary emergency measures quickly evolve into a permanent change in division of labor.

Some cardiac spouses thrive on extra pressure and responsibility. If you're the kind of person who's prone to take care of your mate or if you take pride in being at your best in an emergency, you might welcome the opportunity to take charge. Other spouses feel weary, resentful, and yearn for less pressure and more peace. Any and all of these responses are fine. You just need to know what's actually going on so that you can judge the progress of your recovery and appraise your relationship.

Responsibility and Love

It is natural and appropriate to assume more responsibility during a cardiac crisis. There is nothing more disturbing than seeing someone you love helpless and suffering. You want to do anything and everything you can to help. Cardiac spouses should be awarded a purple heart for bravery for just standing by. Your genuine love and concern for your spouse is expressed when you take charge in a loving and compassionate way.

After Marsh's bypass surgery, he was moved into the intensive care unit. I was thoroughly unprepared for what I witnessed when I first saw him there. Under the huge overhead heating lamp, and attached to several strange-sounding machines and the respirator, Marsh looked like an alien from outer space. He lay very still and his skin felt cold and stiff. He was barely awake, and was receiving morphine for pain.

Marsh had been invaded - to his very core. A half dozen tubes he could not control led in and out of his body. Even his nose and throat had tubes running into them, making it impossible for him to speak. He had no way to say, "Please scratch my nose, it itches." He had no way to let me know that his lips were dry, and that he would appreciate something cool and wet. He had no way to express his fear, anger, or hurt. He had no way to celebrate the fact that he was alive.

I felt immense compassion for him. I chose to be Marsh's protection, his shield. I committed myself to being the buffer between his total vulnerability and the outside world.

We quickly devised a system so that he could communicate. He would write out his questions or statements, tracing one letter at a time with his finger on the sheet at his side. I read his tracing aloud, and when I was correct, he would move on. If not, he would indicate my mistake by raising his index finger, and repeat the letter again. It was a slow process. Sometimes he would forget in the middle of spelling a word and slide into a morphine snooze. (Magic slates or small dry-erase boards and markers should be standard equipment in cardiac care units.)

The first question Marsh traced on the sheet was, "What time is it?" I looked at my watch and told him it was 4:30. He reacted by becoming very upset. His hand returned to the sheet, and he began tracing again. "W-H-A-T D-A-Y? "Through this primitive communication, I began to understand how lost, how helpless, how vulnerable Marsh was. He didn't even know what day it was or how long he had been there. Although it had been a long and difficult day for me too, I vowed to stand there until I couldn't stand anymore, to do what I could for this man I loved so much.

Later the same evening one of the monitoring machines made a new noise, beeping a different message from before. I was asked to step out of the unit, and when I returned Marsh seemed very agitated. Back to the sheet and the letter tracing. One letter at a time, but I got the picture. Marsh had tried to ask the nurse why the machine was making the noise. Her response: "Don't worry about it; you're doing fine." If she had intended to reassure Marsh, she had succeeded in accomplishing the opposite. Being patronized only aggravated his concern.

When the nurse returned, I asked about the sound. She repeated what she'd said to Marsh. I said that I wanted to know. She explained that the machine was reporting a malfunction. Within minutes, the machine was replaced with another that beeped like a familiar friend.

*I was Marsh's shield, his voice, and his protection.
It was necessary . . . and satisfying. The next morning
brought a change. The tubes were removed from his throat,
and he was able to speak for himself.*

As soon as Marsh could talk, my speaking for him
grew insulting. When patients are just out of surgery, or
have just suffered a heart attack, they require total care,
as do newborn children. But just as children gradually
become more independent, cardiac patients rapidly advance from total vulnerability to a level where they are
able to take care of themselves. A parent who takes too
much responsibility fosters dependence, and handicaps
rather than helps a child. The same is true of cardiac
spouses. At each stage of recovery, it's crucial for you to
determine what your mate can and can't handle, relinquishing your responsibility accordingly.

You might be genuinely pleased to see your mate
gradually taking care of his own needs. His increased involvement is a positive sign of recovery. Or you might
experience some ambivalence. Just as some parents find
it hard to let go, you might feel hesitant about stepping
back and letting your spouse fend for himself.

Supporting your mate's recovery means noticing
and encouraging his efforts toward independence. While
you are understandably worried that he might do too
much and have a relapse, do not allow your fear to stand
in the way of his recovery. After witnessing your spouse's
utter helplessness in the hospital, how can you help being overly protective? A cardiac spouse will have some
trouble shifting gears and discovering how much her mate
can realistically handle. Sometimes this causes a serious
problem. One cardiac spouse insisted on spoon-feeding
her husband even though he had been eating without
assistance since the first day after surgery. Another man

imposed mandatory rest periods, even when his wife wasn't tired.

Medical warnings to avoid stress are often misunderstood. Cardiac spouses may "take over" to protect their mates from the danger of undue stress. A most extreme example is the cardiac spouse who forbade her husband to watch television news.

Recovery is an emotional as well as a physical process. Just as you need to continually reassess your idea of your mate's physical progress, you need to review your image of him as a patient. As he becomes stronger, you have to be willing to change your image of yourself, from heroine to helpmate. You must not do everything, only your appropriate share.

If you're afraid to stop overprotecting your mate, remember that heart patients are weaned from total care in a graduated, step-by-step plan by the hospital nursing staff. You can feel confident that he is well enough to function without round-the-clock care and can begin doing things for himself. To help wean cardiac spouses from the patients' bedsides, a hospital where I was invited to be a speaker provides each spouse with a beeper for the duration of the patient's stay. The beeper functions as a symbol of recognition for spouses, since only people important in the recovery process have beepers. There is a practical function as well; wearing a beeper enables cardiac spouses to take better care of themselves during the acute crisis. Cardiac spouses can roam the hospital, take a walk in the fresh air, or even go home for a much-needed nap, and still be in instantaneous contact with the hospital staff.[1]

Maintaining the role of patient or "victim" over the long haul is emotionally destructive and will slow your mate's physical recovery. Encouraging your spouse to remain helpless isn't healthy for either of you. Both of you are in a period of recovery. While your efforts to help are clearly motivated by caring and concern, taking on too much responsibility may ultimately backfire, trapping you into doing more than you should. A combination of rest and some responsibility is the best way for your mate to regain strength and confidence. And your recovery also depends on a shifting balance of power and responsibility.

Responsibility and Fear

The right responsibility is supportive and loving. However, in a cardiac crisis there is the risk of assuming too much responsibility. In this context, *"right" responsibility means basing your actions on an accurate perception of reality.* For example, calling the rescue squad when your mate is having unremitting chest pain is perfectly appropriate. However, calling the doctor every time your spouse looks pale is a sign of over responsibility. Taking on more responsibility than is actually warranted is certainly a sign that fear is making you overreact.

Fear is the number one cause of overresponsibility. Feelings are powerful and fear is no exception. The fear you experience may be out of proportion to the present situation, such as when you're convinced that your mate is on the verge of another heart attack, even though the physician just prescribed more physical activity and less medication.

Cardiac spouses entertain a wide range of exaggerated fears, from losing sleep over one salty pretzel to fantasizing divorce based on an angry outburst.

Your fears may go back to an earlier time when you felt as though you were in danger. When fear is triggered, the feeling is intensified by memories of childhood

- of a time when you were more helpless and dependent. One of the most universal of all human fears is the fear of abandonment. Nearly losing your mate could summon those feelings once again.

Intense fear coupled with the all-consuming sense of responsibility produces an awesome burden, not at all unlike bringing your first newborn home from the hospital. Everything revolves around the baby's schedule and demands. When you're not busy caring for your baby, you worry if he or she is okay. Remember listening intently for the sounds indicating that the baby was still alive after a nap or a night's sleep?

Obviously, your mate is not a totally helpless infant. And you are not totally helpless to cope with your fear of losing your mate. Yet when the fear escalates, you might respond by acting overly responsible, staying awake through most of the night to check your mate's breathing, or waking him up to ask him if he took his medications.

Listening for your partner's breathing is a perfectly normal reaction after all you've been through. But sacrificing your sleep in order to be the permanent night nurse is a sign of deeper, perhaps unfounded fears. When you find your fear overwhelming your sense of realistic responsibility, try the following three techniques to reclaim your balance:

1. Do deep breathing. Sit in an upright chair with your feet on the floor. Focus on following your breath...in and out; don't change your natural breathing rhythm. Imagine that each time you inhale you acquire calm and clarity. Each time you exhale you release fear and overresponsibility. Your body will be unable to hold onto such intense fear as you concentrate on your breath. Continue focused breathing for up to five minutes.

2. Do positive self-talk. Tell yourself that you have a choice about what you say to yourself, what you believe, how you interpret what is happening in your cardiac situation. Here is the perfect opportunity to build and practice solid affirmations that you generate from your qualities of strength and courage. Affirmations should always be worded positively. Use your personal style of language, so you know that the affirmations are yours.

3. Do share with another person. Getting social support is only part of the advantage of talking with another. What rolls around endlessly in your own head continues to gather power. Once exposed to the light of day, what was overwhelming shrinks to a more controllable size. Another person can serve as a reality check, because he is not so intimately affected by the cardiac situation as you are.

SURVIVAL FEARS

If you're like most cardiac spouses, your worst fear is that your mate will die and you will be left alone. Beneath this is the deepest dread: Can you survive that loss? If he dies, how will you go on?

How terrifying to consider the possibility of losing your mate! You may even believe that you can't live without him. But if you search within yourself, you know that you will survive. It may be difficult, painful, and very lonely, but few people actually die of a broken heart. I don't advocate obsession with morbid scenarios. However, you must face your worst fear and believe that you will come out safely on the other side.

Human beings have defense mechanisms to protect them from coping directly with such enormous threats. You are probably unaware of the extent of your terror on a day-to-day basis. The human mechanism devises ways to function even in the face of extreme fear. In order to go about your daily life, you may ignore, rationalize, or deny your fear. But whether or not you're consciously aware of it, your fear manifests itself in a number of ways in your relationship.

The heart-to-heart bond between you and your mate becomes a conduit for unvoiced fears. While you each have unique fears, they reinforce and feed each other's. You may be anxious about your mate coming home from the hospital, doubting your ability to provide adequate care. He senses your insecurity and begins to question whether he's well enough to leave. Once home, you try to limit your spouse's activities so he won't "overdo." Before you know it he's checking his pulse several times a day and expects you to coddle him, convinced that he'd better not strain himself. One spouse, afraid for her husband to leave the security of home, avoided all social activities. She even turned down invitations to their children's homes for Sunday dinner.

Fear makes loving couples turn away from much-needed physical affection. It's typical for cardiac couples to wrongly assume that sexual intercourse is too strenuous to be risked. Many couples pull back without discussing it, each believing that he or she is protecting the other. Your recovering spouse may feel afraid of disappointing you by having less vitality or strength. And after everything you've been told about not "exciting" the patient, it's not easy to relax and enjoy. But physical intimacy can comfort and reassure you. Loss of intimacy does not diminish fear; it may even raise it.

TOO MUCH DEPENDENCE

Heart patients have been known to express fear by acting overly dependent on their mates. What about the patient who wants his spouse to be the only visitor at the hospital? Without even telling her why, he expects his wife to sit in a bedside vigil all day, with no relief from any other visitors. And this behavior may continue once the patient is home. John, an extremely busy account executive with a television station, took off three weeks while his wife had bypass surgery. Well on her way to recovery, his wife continued to fabricate reasons to keep John home from work, and berated him whenever he left the house. Another spouse, Corrine, gave her husband a bell to ring when he needed her so she would be free to move around inside their house. Yet another spouse's frightened husband wouldn't grant her five minutes to do a load of laundry in the basement unless a close relative was nearby. Imagine her frustration, being a prisoner in her own home. In such situations, how can you tell where you end and your spouse begins?

Cardiac patients are naturally preoccupied with their symptoms and emotions. Your mate might cope with his feelings by exhibiting sullen, vociferous, or extremely demanding behavior in a desperate effort to regain control of his life. He may start acting like a prima donna, expecting you to wait on him hand and foot. And you may react by becoming even more focused on your spouse, lavishing extra attention on him, further adapting your life-style to his.

There are a number of areas in which you might assume overresponsibility in a sincere but misguided effort to assist your spouse. You could put yourself in charge of risk factor control, carefully investigating ingredients in foods, or becoming an outspoken advocate of nonsmoking. Gloria proudly described how she protected Milton from stress. She awakened before him, reviewed the morning newspaper and cut out every article she decided was too distressing for him to read. Were there any more than borders to hold on to when Milton opened his paper? How could he feel competent, strong, and whole in relation to Gloria? Some cardiac spouses take on the role of peacemaker and censor all communication among family members in an effort to keep the household stress free. Others become increasingly isolated as they build a life-style centered around their mate's needs instead of their own.

These examples of overdependency remind me of symptoms of addiction. The difference here is that the addiction is to a spouse rather than to a chemical. An addict is a person whose well-being depends on an external source of support and security.[2] You and your mate may be unwittingly involved in an addictive relationship. He needs you to take care of him, and your identity is dependent on providing his care. The longer this cycle continues, the harder it is to break.

My fear that Marsh would die and leave me led to overresponsible behavior that strained our relationship.

Once he was home from the hospital I felt so afraid, so powerless to keep him alive, that I endowed his pills with that power. If he just took every pill, on time, everything would be okay. He would recover. He wouldn't have another heart attack. He wouldn't die.

I reminded him regularly about his medications. It became a routine part of my day to check that he'd taken his pills at the prescribed hour. The fact that he lived through each day was proof that my reminders were working. It never occurred to me that I was interfering. It never crossed my mind that he heard anything but my concern. I never imagined that he resented my questions.

One day, after listening to me go through my litany,

my dear friend Shirley said, "He's a grown man, perfectly capable of monitoring his own medications. Stop nagging. It must be driving him crazy." I was so surprised. I hadn't heard myself nag. I thanked Shirley and went home to undo what by then had become an ingrained responsibility. It was excruciating for several days, like withdrawal from an addiction. It took all my energy to keep quiet, to keep from saying, "Have you taken your pills?"

One morning I came across Marsh's pill box next to the bathroom sink. He had already left for his cardiac rehabilitation class and wouldn't return home until evening. I stood there, paralyzed, wondering whether I should take his pills to him at his class or drive downtown and deliver them to his office. For a brief moment, I fantasized Marsh on the verge of another heart attack. Surely if anything happened it would be my fault. Then I saw how silly that was. I said to myself, "He can take care of himself; it isn't my responsibility." And suddenly the spell was broken. I was free!

I beat the meds, but the real issue was bigger: to break the pattern of dependency that had deepened with Marsh's illness. I needed to deal with my fear, so that we could have an equal relationship, based on mutual dignity and respect.

That night, when Marsh came home, he asked me if I'd noticed that he'd forgotten his pills. I acknowledged seeing the box near the sink, and he said, "It's a good thing I keep an extra day's dose in my desk drawer at the office." Marsh can take care of himself; he can handle the responsibility. I had been overreacting.

When you let your fear get the best of you it can have serious, long-term consequences. Once an isolated type of behavior becomes a habit, it is difficult to change. Recovery doesn't happen overnight or without effort. You must continue to face your fears and look at your actions.

FLEXIBILITY

"Right responsibility" also requires flexibility. In some cases, your mate may remain so incapacitated that you actually need to handle most of the responsibilities. If you are in this position, then the first step is to assess the situation. How much is your mate able to do without your help? What responsibilities are urgent, and which can be set aside? What are the tasks that only you can take care of, and which are the responsibilities that can be shared by friends, relatives, or service providers? The keys to sorting out appropriate responsibility are: assessment, setting priorities, and flexibility.

One cardiac spouse, Rita, described her struggle with right and overresponsibility as a back-and-forth affair. Steve's first heart attack occurred twelve years ago. Just as he was getting back on his feet, he had a second heart attack. Recovery was slow, but Rita gradually resumed her own life, feeling less responsible for Steve's physical care.

Two years ago, Steve's condition deteriorated dramatically. After a third heart attack and congestive heart failure, he is now often mentally confused and requires constant monitoring. Through no fault of her own, Rita is back to doling out medications and assuming responsibility for Steve's physical well-being. She is hungry for her freedom and anxious to give up the role of nurse. Their one ray of hope is that Steve is currently a heart-transplant candidate. In the meantime, Rita's responsibilities continue to shift from day to day.

It's natural to feel resentful when you have to assume an inordinate amount of responsibility, especially over a long period of time. You may feel sad or angry about the time and energy consumed in doing more than your share. And rightfully so. If your mate's condition requires you to take on greater long-term responsibilities, allow yourself to feel the weight of the burden.[3] Pretending to be Superwoman or grumbling under your breath won't help.

Wherever your mate is in the recovery process, you will need to keep reevaluating the situation. By combining flexibility with shared decision making, shifting responsibilities can be a positive part of your relationship.

This Heartmates® comparative checklist will help you to identify the difference between right responsibility and overresponsibility:

HEARTMATES® RESPONSIBILITY CHECKLIST

Right Responsibility	Overresponsibility
Based on reality	An overreaction
Makes you feel calm	Makes you feel panicky
Well thought out	Urgent
Planned	Reckless
Comes from confidence	Motivated by fear
Allows for flexibility	Rigid and uncompromising

The Stress Syndrome

Stress as a risk factor is one of the most misunderstood myths and mysteries of heart disease today. The word alone can send chills of terror up and down your spine. Early in the cardiac crisis, you're given the message *"Don't stress the patient."* The warning is often interpreted as an injunction against sharing worries, concerns, and fears. You stifle your feelings, thinking that you are protecting your mate from stress. You may even take on your mate's worries, trying to lower his stress load by increasing your own.

Your mate is equally sensitive to the stress myth. Stress is one of the most loosely used and least understood words in the English language. Despite the lack of a widely accepted definition of stress, it is universally terrifying to heart patients.

Cardiac patients sometimes use "stress" as an excuse to avoid uncomfortable situations. It isn't unusual to hear a cardiac patient blame or threaten a spouse with some variation of the statement, "Don't raise your voice, you'll make me have another heart attack."

The term "stress" is used generically by many cardiac spouses as well. "I need help coping with stress," is really a call for help in dealing with uncomfortable feelings or for finding appropriate avenues of expression or relief. Physical outlets that help people relax are often termed "stress reducers." Running, or any type of exercise, therapeutic massage, and warm baths are activities recommended to help the cardiac spouse reduce stress.

Dr. Robert Eliot's attempts to solve the mysteries of stress and its relationship to heart disease have been inconclusive. He maintains that while everyone of us knows, or thinks he knows, what stress is, each person experiences stress in a highly individual way.[4]

Another problem in defining stress is that it affects different people in different ways. Four weeks after her heart attack, Julie felt frustrated because her doctor hadn't given her permission to drive her car. It was stressful to depend on someone else to chauffeur her around. But the thought of driving by herself also made her anxious. She was reluctant to ask her doctor when she could resume driving, fearful that his answer would verify her worst fear: a permanent life-style of severely limited freedom and mobility.

Dr. Hans Selye's definitive book, *The Stress of Life*, considers the question of whether stress factors in the environment actually produce harmful effects. His findings reinforce the idea that stress is a necessary part of a person's life.[5]

What stress is and how it works to our benefit or harm is not yet clear. Despite this, cardiac recovery decisions are often based on the myths. When physicians or cardiac patients make long-range decisions based on an assessment of stress level, they are dealing with a complex subject, with largely unknown consequences.

The notion that a stress-free life is a more meaningful or qualitatively better life is another myth. Eliminating stress from a cardiac patient's life is impossible. And creating and living in a controlled environment, totally devoid of stimulus or conflict, makes for a boring and meaningless existence. A certain amount of stress is necessary to remain vital. Dr. Selye contends that,"Life without stress is death."

Michael, a minister of a large congregation for twenty-five years, had a heart attack. On the advice of his physician, he retired from his beloved calling because the work was too stressful. He has become increasingly depressed and apathetic, wandering around at home like a captain without a ship. Between income from Nancy's work as a medical technician and a pension Michael receives from the national office of their church, they are able to make ends meet. But financial security doesn't resolve the stress of the loss Michael has sustained: the loss of meaningful work and the ability to make a contribution to his community.

Who can say which is more stressful: to practice ministry, feeling needed and helpful, but heavily stressed by the demanding nature of the work, or to be a depressed pensioner, whose life stress is minimal? What are the consequences of Nancy reversing roles to become the major breadwinner and Michael being stripped of his life's calling?

Michael and Nancy's case clearly indicates that the complexity of each unique cardiac situation must be assessed if good recommendations and decisions about emotional stress and its effects are going to be made.

The setting of physical limitations is a different and separate issue. A "stress test" determines a safe level of physical activity, and should be heeded as a guide for healthy levels of physical exertion. When a patient's work is physical in nature, stress test results may indicate necessary reductions in work. They also serve an important role in medical diagnosis and provide progress reports for the patient.

What about the stress that already exists at home? Both of you may be pointing fingers at each other, blaming the patient's rising blood pressure on each other's bad habits.

The condition of your marital relationship may add stress to an already volatile situation. The family is a complex system, made more vulnerable by today's social changes and fast pace. In a crisis, each of you is more likely to be impatient and intolerant. Fear and anxiety cause you to be more irritable so that things you used to be able to accept and ignore suddenly seem like a big deal. Try not to judge the quality of your marriage in the midst of a crisis. It wasn't perfect before, why should all the problems magically disappear now?

If you are lucky, your marriage is a support system and a haven. Probably, though, there are times when it is a source of comfort and other times when being with each other intensifies the stress. Even if it seems as if your marriage is the main source of stress in your life, keep in mind that the familiarity and continuity it provides is an important anchor during what would otherwise be a chaotic period. And remember; this is a time to be especially gentle and understanding with each other.

From Caring to Caretaking

A great deal of your time and energy is devoted to looking after the needs of your recovering mate. One reason that you've taken on so much responsibility is because you care. But that's not the only reason. There is "caretaking." Just as there is a distinction between right responsibility and overresponsibility, caring and caretaking are two different things.

Helplessness is the primary feeling behind caretaking behavior. Helplessness is an assault on your sense of power. When you see your spouse vulnerable or in pain, you feel helpless. You wish that you could do something to fix it. Since there is nothing you can do to change the reality of your mate's heart disease, you compensate for your feelings by taking control.

Consider the cardiac spouse whose mate refuses to quit smoking. Everyone knows that smoking is high on the list of risk factors for heart disease. Each cigarette adds to your growing fear of losing your mate. You feel the pain and sadness that goes with watching your spouse self-destruct. You may nag, cajole, beg, even get angry and accusatory to try to get him to quit. Nothing works.

In fact, *you are helpless!* Attempting to control the uncontrollable inevitably leads to an image of yourself as a failure.

Women in our culture learn early to be caretakers. Beginning at a young age, girls are rewarded for being sensitive to other people's feelings; by maturity they may be unable to recognize their own. When asked, many adult women find it impossible to know or say what they need. Consequently, their needs are suppressed or denied.

As much as women today may be resentful or rebellious about being caretakers, we tend to fall into this familiar role when we are in crisis. Being a caretaker provides the illusion of control, masks helplessness, and keeps us from getting our own needs met.

Your image of yourself also contributes to your tendency to be a caretaker. The stereotype of the "good woman" or the "little woman" is a portrait of a gentle, sweet, even-tempered, and, inherently, long-suffering woman. Many women have been conditioned to strive for this ideal, and they struggle to maintain such a picture of themselves, even during a crisis. Everything is at risk, and the only tools the "good woman" has at hand are sweetness and a willingness to suffer for "her man." She doesn't recognize her own feelings. She doesn't know she has needs or that in order for her to recover from her crisis she needs to take care of herself. She has been granted no permission to express her resentment about having to care for a mate who may not be caring for himself. Or worse, she may be caring for a mate who is *only* caring about himself.

If you take responsibility for your mate's feelings, activities, and his life, he will become dependent and you will become resentful. The "good woman" continues to maintain a sweetness that tastes bitter, and caretaking that has lost its foundation of caring.

It is a commonly held premise that the heart patient's recovery is in the hands of his spouse. It isn't! However irrational, you may feel personally responsible for your mate's health, recovery, and even his life. But you're not! *You didn't cause his heart disease, and you can't cure it.*

Expressing your caring, rather than becoming a

caretaker, requires a delicate balance. No one can make another person change. You are helpless to do anything that can make your spouse take his illness seriously. Sometimes cardiac spouses use blame or shame in an effort to coerce their mates to quit smoking, eat carefully, take medications religiously, exercise regularly, and eliminate unnecessary stress. Many cardiac patients are admitted "workaholics" and may strongly resist changing or limiting their careers in response to their heart condition.

Your caretaking may be in direct proportion to your husband's denial. The more he pushes himself, the more you nag him to slow down. If he makes a joke about eating prime rib, you counter with a lecture on the evils of cholesterol. You tend to interpret anything less than perfection and instant reversal of decades-long habit as denial or irresponsibility. If his attitude reflects a lack of concern for his condition, you double your efforts, and exhaust yourself on his behalf.

The same is true when it comes to feelings. In our culture it is more acceptable for women to have and express feelings than it is for men. Up to now, heart disease has been principally a male disease. It is customary for male heart patients to ignore or deny their feelings of anger or sadness. Men also have learned to mask their fear with bravado. Over many years, you and your mate's emotions have become so intertwined that you may unconsciously take on his unexpressed feelings.

At one time or another, you've probably said, "I'm carrying the weight of the world on my shoulders," or, "I'm worrying for both of us." There's real danger in assuming your mate's feelings. You can't carry the burden without exacting a cost to yourself. The consequence is your sense of failure, depression, even despair. Your genuine concern and desire to protect your mate will ultimately backfire, resulting in the opposite effect. If your mate doesn't have to deal with his own feelings, he can't recover from the emotional dimension of his cardiac crisis. The greater your fear, the more the patient pushes himself, ignoring prescribed physical limitations. The more you express concern about heart-healthy diet, the more stubborn he gets, refusing to give up fatty foods.

Caring about your mate doesn't mean doing everything for him at the expense of your own needs. And genuine caring involves letting go and encouraging your mate's independence.

Ultimately, it is not your responsibility to *make* your spouse recover. You can help. You can be supportive. And you can care. *But you do not have the power to save his life.* No person can take that basic responsibility for another.

From Patient to Partner

There are negative consequences of acting in an overresponsible way. Getting stuck in the rigid role of caretaker fosters dependency, which, in turn, may slow the physical recovery of your mate.

Many years ago the treatment for a heart attack was weeks, sometimes months, of bed rest. The most up-to-date information suggests that lying in bed weakens rather than strengthens patients. Muscles that aren't used tend to atrophy. Today, cardiac patients are encouraged to begin walking two or three days after a heart attack or after surgery.

Cardiac rehabilitation programs are based on a carefully modulated regimen of activity interspersed with rest. Trying to limit your spouse's physical activity by doing everything for him directly opposes modern medical wisdom.

When you take too much responsibility for your mate you also hamper your own recovery. If you're continually taking care of him, you are probably not taking good enough care of yourself. And encouraging your mate's dependence can be psychologically and emotionally damaging to both of you.

Finally, attitude has a tremendous impact on recovery. Cardiac patients struggle with the challenge of holding on to their self-respect. Perception of self-worth can be negatively affected by the stigma associated with heart disease. Rebuilding a healthy self-image happens gradually, as your mate successfully handles more and more, and integrates realistic limitations.

A positive attitude takes motivation and confidence. If you persist in taking over for your mate, he may start to wonder if his condition is more serious than he's been told. Doing things for him that he's capable of doing for himself makes him feel handicapped and inadequate. In response to all the "help" he received from his spouse, one patient reported, "It's as if having a heart attack curdled my brain." After a while, an individual who sees himself as an invalid will begin to believe that he is truly "in-valid." No cardiac spouse wants to contribute to such a negative attitude.

Trapped in a situation of overresponsibility and caretaking is no way to meet either of your recovery needs. Both of you may be strained in a relationship that needs caring, not caretaking, and right responsibility, not overresponsibility. Stress levels in the relationship may have escalated. Both of you may feel smothered; neither feels supported.

If you feel that you're doing well sharing and balancing responsibilities, congratulate yourself! If not, the following five steps can help you start shifting responsibilities in a way that will enhance and strengthen your relationship.

HEARTMATES® FIVE-STEP PLAN FOR RIGHT RESPONSIBILITY

Step 1: Accept your powerlessness. This is easier said than done, but it is the critical first step. Until you can accept that caretaking and controlling are running your life, you will be shortsighted and your perceptions will be distorted. Continuous attempts at managing the unmanageable will lead you to a dead end.

Step 2: Assess your situation realistically. You know more about your situation than any expert or outsider. Be realistic about what responsibilities are urgent, and which ones can be put aside. Don't downplay or overdramatize the seriousness of your situation.

Step 3: Look honestly at your own behavior. Without blame or self-deprecation, analyze what you are doing and evaluate the positive and negative consequences to you, to your mate, and to your marriage.

Step 4: Differentiate between right and overresponsibility, caring and caretaking. You may want to discuss steps three and four with your spouse or a confidante you trust, to help you determine these differences.

Step 5: Make changes. The direction of change should be relative to where you are in recovery. As time passes, and you move farther away from the acute period of physical care, you need to begin to shift your attention from your mate's health to your own. Your recovery reestablishes your sense of self-worth and well-being, and opens you to real intimacy.

Wean yourself from the responsibility of being available for any and every demand. As the weeks and months go by, it is necessary to return to other aspects of life. At first the change may be small: leaving the house for a short time to do some shopping or take clothes to the cleaners. The next separate excursion may be lunch with a friend, a concert, or community meeting. It may be advisable to build up to a bigger separation, like taking a retreat weekend, or visiting one of your grown children for a few days.

These steps are part of your recovery process. They take time, effort, commitment, and courage. No change comes easily. Lifelong habits conditioned by early training and cultural acceptance are very difficult to change.

Don't underestimate the healing power of sharing these issues with others who are in similar straits. Find someone you trust to cheer you on. Celebrate as you take steps to further your personal recovery.

CHAPTER NOTES

1. Bishop Clarkson Hospital in Omaha, Nebraska, has put this creative idea into practice - their cardiac spouses are fortunate indeed.
2. Stanton Peele and Archie Brodsky, *Love and Addiction* (New York: New American Library, 1975), p. 6.
3. In *Mainstay: For The Well Spouse of the Chronically Ill*, Maggie Strong gives the well spouse permission to feel bad about, resent, even hate, without guilt, the

unchosen burden of responsibility when a partner becomes chronically ill.

I have been fortunate to have the opportunity to learn from William J. Doherty, Ph.D. (co-author of *Families and Health and Medical Family Therapy*) in a variety of professional settings. His groundbreaking work envisions collaborative healthcare systems staffed by professionals who respect and acknowledge the needs and difficulties of spouses who have assumed the role of caregiver in families organized around a chronic illness. His ethical stance emphasizes factoring in every one's needs to achieve the goals of agency (autonomy) and communion (interpersonal connection) for the family.

4. Robert Eliot, M.D., *Stress and the Major Cardiovascular Disorders* (Mt. Kisco, NY: Futura Publishing Co., 1979), p. 14.

5. Hans Selye, M.D., *The Stress of Life* (New York: McGraw Hill Book Co., 1956), p. 299. See appendix E in this book for an essay on stress written by massage therapist and health educator, Pamela R.Borgmann, RN, M.Th.

Does Time Heal All Wounds?

My sense of my own identity was permanently changed when I became a cardiac spouse. I stopped believing that I had complete control over my life and my destiny. Marsh has heart disease. There is nothing I can do to alter that fact. I live in a world of imperfection, where change beyond my control occurs instantaneously.

I lost my innocence. Before Marsh's heart attack, I lived life as if it were an exciting adventure. I believed there were no limits to what Marsh and I could accomplish together. In one shocking moment, my naiveté was gone. Eventually a new reality was born in its place. I am neither invincible nor limitless. I am human.

I let go of my subconscious belief in immortality. Marsh's brushes with death made me realize that our time on earth is limited, that we will not live forever. I had been squandering time as if I had eternity in my back pocket. I experience time differently now, treasuring each day, and I have learned to set my priorities more thoughtfully.

My beliefs and dreams were gone. My wounds were so deep, I hurt to my very core. My pain has diminished with time. Still, I'm sometimes reminded of it all when I look in the mirror and see the lines in my face or the sadness in my eyes.

Coping with heart disease is a pervasive, enduring, and lifelong process. The original trauma may be past, but there are permanent changes. Your body, mind, and spirit have been scarred.

Fortunately, time is on your side. Your mate has survived and so have you. As the weeks and months pass, you are reassured more and more that life goes on. Time has taught you a number of things. You're no longer afraid to leave your mate at home, and you are less involved with his physical symptoms. You've come through the crisis with increased strength, resiliency, and adaptability.

But your journey isn't over. Everything has changed, and even time can't make things "normal" again. You cannot erase what has happened. Our cultural conditioning perpetuates the myth that if you just do everything right, all will be fine; your pain will vanish and you'll live happily ever after. But you're not living a fairy tale; this is your life. There is no magic that can make the recent past disappear. There are no pills or time machines to transport you back to an earlier time of innocence. The cardiac spouse faces countless disappointments, a suddenly altered future, and broken dreams.[1] Your spouse's heart disease has affected your life-style, your financial security, your marital relationship, your most deeply held beliefs, your very identity.

You now question everything: your values, ideas, and convictions, even who you are. If you have always believed that your husband is stronger than you, his physical weakness and vulnerability caused by heart disease threaten this belief. If you've measured your intimacy by the degree of passion in your sexual relationship, new limitations may make you reevaluate your perceptions. Firmly held ideas, such as, "Nothing bad can happen if you believe in God," or, "These things happen to other people," are now meaningless, and you feel confused and betrayed. The cardiac crisis has upset your security and shattered your most precious dreams. Something is very, very wrong. You have reached that universal and dramatic realization that *nothing will ever be the same.*

Confrontation with permanent change can be devastating. Heart disease exacts its costs: limited activity, lost security, and painful adjustments in your personal relationships. Your feelings of sadness and anger are valid, whether they are in reaction to something small, like giving up your favorite foods, or more profound, like relinquishing long-term plans for the future.

Being a cardiac spouse forces you to remove your rose-colored glasses. Your mate's heart disease has brought you face to face with your own personal reality. Included in that reality are wounds from losses. You've lost deeply valued things in your work, recreational, private, and family life; in your routine and life-style; and in your heart of hearts, where your long-held dreams, values, and priorities reside.

There is no cure for heart disease. What has happened is irreversible and permanent. Who can say why you and your spouse have had to cope with heart disease? The reasons are not always apparent; perhaps focusing on "why" only distracts you from the challenge that change provides. All change is difficult, but not universally negative.

But just as there is no end without a beginning, there is no loss without the hope of gain. In this case, there is a positive path to traverse and a chance for personal healing and growth. Wisdom of the ages includes the Tao definition of crisis as "opportunity" and Hippocrates's perception, "Healing is a matter of time, but it is sometimes also a matter of opportunity."[2] *Carpe diem.* In our time, no one has advocated better for hope, healing, and humor than Norman Cousins, whose view was that, "Healing is possible, even when curing is not."[3]

Grief and Loss

Human life implies death and loss. Perhaps one of the most difficult things we face is learning how to absorb and survive loss - how to "let go."

Although grief is usually part of the emotional process following a death, it pertains to all change. Every change we experience has two elements, loss and potential gain. *Grief* is the word in our language that describes human reactions to loss. To adapt to the losses accompanying heart disease, you may need to grieve for your past, your life as it was before the cardiac crisis.

The pains that are part of the grieving process are many and diverse.[4] Having dealt with one pain it is often a surprise and disappointment to find that down the road there is another, unrelated pain that envelops the wounded. You may hurt as you become aware that you have experienced a devastating loss, and need to make the effort to persevere, to survive. Then there is the pain of longing and the loneliness for the old life before the losses. The related need is to maintain and honor the memory of what was. Yet another pain is the pain of vulnerability, and the need is to be held in love, embraced as a child is by a loving parent. Then there is the mental pain of not understanding. The intellectual mind needs to understand the loss in order to come to acceptance, to establish meaning in what may seem meaningless. And there is the pain that is hunger for significance, the human need to make something good come out of tragedy.

The custom of mourning is as old as life itself. Our human cultural past is rich with wisdom. The original

Sanskrit definition of mourning means "remembering." In Greek, mourning means "caring." Mourning really includes both components. Centuries ago, the rabbis of Judea codified rituals of mourning. The first year after a loss was divided into smaller parts: the first week, the first month, and the first eleven months. Observances and rituals for each period were defined, giving the family permission to mourn and providing a guide for "working through" grief.

And the present, too, is rich with wisdom. "For mourning is the constant reawakening that things are now different."[5] The Yakima Indian Nation gives us: "Mourning makes peace with change."[6] In order to work through your grief you must acknowledge and express the feelings generated by loss. You also need to "tell your story" and talk about your struggle in order to understand what has happened. Remembering and caring enable you to integrate and accept the loss.

Elisabeth Kübler-Ross, whose monumental work lifted the cultural taboo of silence about loss and death, suggested stages through which mourners pass, progressing from shock, disbelief, denial, and numbness through anger and depression toward acceptance.[7] Her analysis legitimized the process of grieving for many. People don't necessarily experience the stages in order; some move back and forth from stage to stage. Others experience several stages simultaneously. Even mourners who have reached the stage of acceptance may continue at times to wrestle with fears and yearn for the past.

Although professional literature has established the validity and therapeutic value of grief, there is still social pressure to keep the mourning responses brief. We are a people journeying in the fast lane, intolerant of anything that takes longer than the speed of light. Our culture adds to our burden and undermines our self-esteem by ignoring and avoiding the individual's *normal* need to grieve losses. Despite pressure to "hurry up and get on with life," it's essential to allow yourself time and attention to mourn. You may be at your most vulnerable, but you need to proceed through grief at your own pace, without a model, a guide, or unqualified support.

The cardiac spouse's losses are real and important, albeit intangible, invisible to others, neither legitimized by society nor voiced by you.[8] If you don't allow yourself to grieve, you will get stuck in a psychological rut. Resisting the natural process may result in physical consequences, in illness. Research has shown that natural immunity is reduced when someone experiences sudden and intense change; grieving people are more susceptible to disease for up to two years after a crisis. And you'll be bereft of the seeds born from grieving and necessary to plant a new crop of realistic dreams for the garden of your future.

Once you acknowledge that the cardiac crisis has wounded you, you can begin to look at your losses in earnest. Remember that your purpose is to heal and adapt from what *was* to what *is*.

The Healing Process

Healing requires time, but our culture is impatient. If your wounds were obvious, involving a scar or crutches, friends and family would better understand your need to take the time to heal. But your wounds are invisible. Judging by your surface appearance, everyone assumes that you are doing just fine. And in some ways, you are. But you still may be struggling to accept the permanent changes brought on by heart disease. Even if it means going against the grain, you need to permit yourself time to heal.

Healing is highly individual. Each person has individual needs and timing. Treat yourself kindly. Don't pressure yourself to rush through this. Don't push yourself faster than you can go, and don't let others, uncomfortable or impatient with your pace, pressure you into activities or decisions for which you're not yet ready.

Time is central to the healing process. But it alone isn't enough. You must also be willing to cleanse your wounds: to confront your losses and rage, and to mourn in order to come to terms with the reality of your life now. Forgiveness makes it possible to accept your imperfection, your spouse's, and the uncontrollable events that have happened. And the final step in healing is to turn from the process of introspection to reconnect with the world around you and look forward with anticipation as your present becomes the future.

Whether you are recovering from the trauma of chronic illness or the finality of death, the process of grief and healing is essentially the same. There are five basic steps in healing:

1. Recognizing and naming your wounds
2. Facing reality
3. Releasing your feelings
4. Updating your images
5. Forgiveness

Recognizing Your Wounds

It's natural to try to escape pain. One way is to ignore what's happened. In some respects, that's easy to do. If your mate has had a full physical recovery, he may look healthier than he has in years. Recovered bypass patients often have ruddy complexions and report that they "feel great." A regular exercise program has probably made your spouse physically fit and more active than he was before his heart attack.

Some cardiac spouses try to avoid pain by trivializing it. You may tell yourself, "This is no big deal," and attempt to live your life exactly as before. Other cardiac spouses are afraid of self-pity, continually asking, "What in the world have I got to complain about?" and denying themselves permission to examine very real wounds.

Where you are in the life cycle when heart disease hits is a critical component determining the scope and depth of your pain. Young cardiac couples will face the pain and strain of deciding whether to have a family, or even whether to stay together. Not many years later, the pain of heart disease may be complicated because of child-rearing issues, and having the responsibility of children and adolescents who also experience the pain of a parent's heart disease. Older couples, having sacrificed for family, will experience the pain of broken dreams. Heart disease cheats them out of their leisure years, a time they believed would be restful or adventurous, and free from responsibility.

Trying to escape pain only sends it underground. Wounds need fresh air to heal. Like an infection, pain continues to run its course, and cannot be cured with a Band-Aid or the casual pretense that it doesn't exist.

Denying reality won't help you heal. Denial hinders the recovery process and diminishes your freedom and spontaneity. An extreme, but not unusual, example involves Marilyn, the fifty-one-year-old wife of a cardiac bypass patient. Marilyn proudly described how she avoided her own painful feelings regarding Robert's surgery. She worked out a plan so that she would never see his scars. The last thing she wanted was to be reminded of the nightmare they'd been through. She made sure to be out of the bedroom when he was dressing or undressing. She got into bed only after Robert had turned out the light, so she wouldn't see his bare chest. If Robert went to sit by their apartment-house pool in his swimming trunks, Marilyn would find something to do that kept her inside. This carefully wrought plan required more and more of Marilyn's energy and attention. What began as a solution ended up being a trap. Instead of diminishing her pain, Marilyn found that her life was dictated by her denial.

Recognizing your wounds may be difficult for several reasons, starting with the fact that you weren't raised to identify and value your own needs. You may be so conditioned to the role of caretaker that you honestly don't know that you have been hurt. A successful caretaker puts in twenty-four-hour days and every effort to take care of others and combat the inevitable. The caretaker doesn't know how to assess her own needs. She has been given no permission to let down or let go; the way *she* feels is the least of her worries. She's always on duty, perennially cheerful, and indefatigable, even after years of service.

But what will happen when you move beyond denial and habit to confront that deep and universal fear of the unknown? Will you survive if you remove the Band-Aids and see your wounds? Will you drown in your tears, or will they be a relief and a comfort? What proof is there that, if you look at what is lost, outdated, or gone, you will rise out of despair and chaos to something secure and meaningful?

Fear of the unknown can be fought only with faith and courage. You will never achieve peace of mind unless you come to terms with reality.

> Courage is the price that life exacts
> for granting peace.
> The souls that know it not,
> know no release from little things.[9]

Recognizing your wounds does not guarantee positive growth. But if you have the faith that there is something beyond your pain and the courage to act in the face of your fear, you will be closer to an acceptance of your reality.

Your pain is symptomatic of the losses you've experienced. *There is no way around pain; you must go through it.* Pain's partner, vulnerability, opens the door so you can look at yourself and your life. If you use all your energy to keep the door tightly shut, you will not heal. Your wounds will continue to fester and ooze, and your life will become more and more constricted with each passing month. You may never again have such an opportunity to evaluate your life, to name and acknowledge your losses, to take charge of what you want and need in the present, to focus your energy on achieving new and realistic goals.

Facing Reality

The second step in the process of healing is discerning what your loss means to you. A wound can heal only after its severity is determined. You must think about what has happened before you can figure out how you can heal.

One of the best ways to understand something is to name it, to talk about it. Seek out friends who will listen to you. Plan outings, like lunch in the back booth at your favorite restaurant or a secluded walk by the lake or in the woods, where you can talk undisturbed.

To fully grasp what you have lost, *review* (re-view) and *relive* your experience - it's an integral part of grieving. (See appendix B, Self-help Tools, for the Evening Review, which is particularly useful to the cardiac spouse because it provides a review structure. Reviewing is a mental activity that helps a person to think clearly, see reality, and establish order in the chaos of the crisis.)

Begin at the beginning. Tell a friend *your* story, what happened to you, how you felt and feel. Each time you relate it, your story will change.

Psychologist Shelley Taylor has done extensive research linking recovery with people's ability to tell their stories.[10] Her studies indicate that, "...tragedy brings forth the need to create meaning - to tell new stories - that can reweave the frayed ends of life into a coherent whole." As you try to understand, you may find that you need to get straight facts and information you have lost. Contact the doctor, family members, or anyone who might have the information you've missed or forgotten. Reviewing your experience helps you separate the reality of what has happened from your feelings about what happened. Keep talking. Over a period of time it will become clear to you how your life has changed.

As you talk, you'll begin to explore important questions that help you test what is real:

- How does my spouse's heart condition really affect me?
- What is most important now in my life?
- What's realistic for me to expect of myself now?
- How do I feel about the ways in which our relationship has changed?

You need to lay a foundation for constructing a new, more

realistic image of yourself. It helps, when you are testing what is real, to share your thoughts and ideas with a trusted friend who will listen and can respond in ways that deepen or broaden your perspective.

Releasing Feelings

Facing reality uncovers your feelings. At this point in the process, you begin to feel the sadness, pain, and anger associated with your losses. You may feel overwhelmed or out of control. But the pain of knowing is also cleansing. If you've been unable to cry since all this began, your tears may come now. Imagine them washing and cleansing your wounds; they offer relief, a loving gift to yourself. If you can, allow yourself to cry with someone you trust, who can give you support.

The release of emotion, through words and tears, helps heal your wounds. This may be an appropriate time to seek professional help. A skilled therapist can give you support, help you test reality, and listen to you.

Another release is writing. Keep a journal and use it to communicate with yourself. Set aside time every day to sit in a safe and comfortable place, tune into your thoughts and feelings, and write in your journal.

Remember, *everyone who experiences loss grieves.* Your feelings indicate how deeply affected you are by your losses. Be aware of and accept your need to grieve; honor yourself and your life.

Many people believe that the outward expression of feelings is a sign of weakness. I contend that the opposite is true. It requires the utmost courage to express your feelings, and only the strong dare to do so. Shakespeare's advice in *Macbeth* applies to cardiac spouses today:

"Give sorrow words; the grief that does not speak
Whispers the o'er fraught heart and bids it break."[11]

Anger may be the most difficult emotion for you to
acknowledge, and its strength one of the surprises related
to your partner's cardiac crisis. Facing and paying attention to anger may feel to you like the first fatal step on
the road to total disintegration. You tell yourself you can't
risk that, because you have to stay strong to care for your
spouse and family.

Some cardiac spouses don't feel entitled to their
anger. You weren't widowed by heart disease, so you have
no right to be angry, you think. You may feel ashamed
admitting to yourself that you have anger. One cardiac
spouse told me that anger was a sin. When you feel wrong
for being angry, even acknowledging it can prompt a sense
of unworthiness and low self-esteem.

Why bother with anger when it's so difficult? Why
not sidestep it, accept and forgive? Because it's not possible! Anger is a normal human response to hurt and loss.
You can't reach acceptance without first dealing with your
anger.

In order to let go of your anger, you must stop holding on to it, protecting it, and hiding it from yourself and
others. Your anger may take the form of blame; you might
blame the doctor, the professional staff, even the hospital system for how you feel or what's happened to you or
your spouse. Your anger might be directed against your
spouse for having heart disease, for smoking, for being a
"type A," or even for the genetic factors he inherited.
Maybe you're letting your anger smolder, resenting how
your mate has treated you. It's conceivable that you feel
angry and hurt that your mate has withdrawn since all of
this began. Perhaps you feel emotionally deprived, sorely
in need of care and affection. Or maybe you are furious

that your spouse has not appreciated your extra effort on his behalf over these months.

If you were to express your feelings to your spouse, you might be amazed at how your perceptions differ. Even if you disagree, you still have acknowledged and named your anger. Your anger is based on *your* perception of your experience. You don't need to be fair, accurate, or unselfish. Holding on to your anger because you don't think it is "justified" will isolate you and add to the emotional distance between you and your mate. Sheltered anger also builds walls, shutting out friends' understanding and support.

Wives who relied on their faith before the cardiac crisis may find themselves angry at God. Helen, who had been very religious, felt as though God had turned His back on her. Another cardiac spouse, Caroline, described how unfair it was for God to abandon her after she had "been good" all her life. Yet another spouse believed that God was punishing her with the cardiac crisis.

People who live their faith, trusting their relationship with God, can afford to express their anger in words and tears. They don't need to keep their anger hidden inside. People abandon God by withholding their anger; by expressing it, they discover that God has been there for them all along.

Release of feelings doesn't happen in a day or a week; the process occurs over time and in small measures. You may hesitate to release feelings, certain that doing so will be overpowering. That is rarely the case. Your psyche, naturally healing itself, will determine a safe pace.

For a while, I went along acting as if everything were okay. I felt numb as I went through the motions of my everyday life and routine. I forced myself to stay calm, managing the household, the kids, and myself as steadily as I could. Protected by my robot-like efficiency, I told myself I was fine. I was perfectly capable of handling what had happened.

I had been warned that Marsh needed rest and no stress in order to heal. How could I tell him that I was afraid he would be disabled or die? How could I tell him that I was afraid he would never work again, that I was frozen with anxiety about money for our family's future? How could I tell him that I was infuriated at him for not taking better care of his body and for causing me all this distress? How could I tell him that my trust was eroded, now that he had proved he was not immortal and invincible? How could I tell him how scared I was that he would keel over and die if he was late or missed his pills? How could I tell him that I was waking up in the middle of the night to listen for his breath, scared he was lying dead beside me? How could I tell him that I was afraid to leave the house, sure that his life was my responsibility, and that I hated it?

Of course I didn't say these things, at least not aloud, to Marsh or to anyone. I was ashamed of my feelings and kept them hidden inside, becoming progressively more isolated and alone. Instead of expressing my fear, I concentrated on my competence. I repaired the back fence with a hammer and nails. I busily painted our bedroom and wallpapered our bathroom. I never once considered how Marsh felt, lying in bed recovering as I frantically painted us into separate corners.

Life became a series of mechanical actions without meaning. Like a coronary artery slowly closing down, the life and love between us got so sluggish it was barely enough to keep our relationship alive.

It was many months later that the incongruity of my behavior hit me. Here I was, acting as if I didn't need Marsh, when there was no one in the world I treasured more. I was so terrified of losing him that I was pushing him away. Instead of drawing near, I had constructed a wall of bravado between us, trying desperately to prove that I could live without the one person I loved most. After feeling so betrayed, I was determined never to be that vulnerable again. I had decided that if there was a chance of Marsh's abandoning me, I would leave first, if not physi-

cally, then emotionally.

A wave of shame went through me as I realized what I had done. How could I be so selfish? Marsh had been sick and needed me, and I had been concerned only with protecting myself. Like a waterfall, tears began to stream down my face. They washed away my shame, and I forgave myself. Having released the pain, I made a new and conscious vow to share my love and vulnerability, to be Marsh's heartmate.

Acknowledging what is gives you the raw material for a new start. With acceptance, you can see how the cardiac crisis has affected you. Ventilated sorrow and anger melt away and new compassion toward your mate and yourself emerges. You can't change what has already happened, neither can you turn back time, but once you've faced reality, grieved, and cleansed your wounds, you can move ahead.

The Power of Images

Trust is based on a series of experiences that provide a reliable image of reality. Whether you're aware of it or not, you probably trust the security of your life-style, a stable relationship with your mate, and your expectations of the future. As each day dawns, and everything you take for granted in your life continues to be there, your images are supported and reinforced. Until something happens to threaten your images, you continue to place your trust in the world view you've created.

All cardiac spouses share a loss of trust as our images shatter with the unexpected shock of heart disease. We need to repair our images to complete the process of healing. In the adult world, images are rarely discussed or taken seriously. Images are considered to be the product of children's imaginations, or of the senility of the aged, or the delusions of the mentally disabled.

Imagery is a combination of our mental and emotional perceptions of events. We believe that the world is the way we "see" it. Beyond conscious awareness, our minds and emotions interpret and define reality. Thus our images form the basis of our world view and are the foundation of our actions. We trust our images. *We respond to our images as if they were reality.*

If your image of the hospital is of a place with a competent and caring staff, you will feel satisfied with the quality of care your spouse receives. If your image of the hospital is of a place of helplessness and isolation, that may give rise to a very different interpretation: that it's an impersonal, untrustworthy place. The truth is probably somewhere in between, but your image is *your* reality.

The power of imagery and of the mind-matter connection are not well understood, but even the superstitious are familiar with the concept of a self-fulfilling prophecy: the idea that what we imagine eventually comes to pass. A patient overheard staff describing him as "the man with the galloping heart." This is a severe and debilitating condition, yet this patient continued to thrive. Some years later he explained to his doctor that he attributed his amazing recovery to the fact that he had a galloping heart, which he believed meant a robust and rugged heart that would not fail him. Overhearing the prognosis that his bypass repair was probably "good for five years" may have imprinted an image that had a physical effect on another cardiac patient. Exactly five years later he returned to surgery for a second bypass.

On the positive side, there has been research that indicates that when patients make the effort to construct and then believe positive images, using the technique of visualization to "see" chemicals or rays destroying all the cancer cells in the body, for example, they may actually live longer than patients whose imagery is negative.[12]

Programs designed to reverse heart disease are as yet statistically positive with only very small samples, but cardiac patients who *participate* in their recovery, actively involving themselves in a food plan or exercise program, or yoga and meditation, or walking regularly in their local shopping center, and who *believe* that they are promoting their good health, experience an enhanced quality of life.

Norman Cousins, author, healer, and heart patient, described walking on a golf course and seeing medics from an ambulance rush to the aid of a man who had suddenly collapsed. The medical personnel were monitoring his blood pressure and pulse. Cousins read the monitor, but seeing that the man looked really scared, put his hand on the patient's shoulder and told him that he had a very strong heart and was going to make it. Within a minute's time the monitor's dangerously high reading had returned to almost normal.[13]

If imagery has power in the physical realm, it seems indisputable that it would affect psychological and spiritual health as well.

Penny, age thirty-two, sat weeping on a park bench as she watched her two toddlers playing enthusiastically on the swings. She cried because she believed she had lost the dream of what she called a "normal" family. She grieved because her family could not live carelessly or worry free, now that her husband had heart disease. Her children would no longer be innocent offspring of perfectly healthy parents.

In Penny's mind, the image of an ideal family precluded serious illness and pain. Her ability to cry and her willingness to discuss her lost image were encouraging signs of recovery. As she expressed her feelings of disappointment and frustration, she began to redefine what "normal" might mean, and to rebuild her image of her family's future.

A crisis forces us to focus on what's real. When we hold our images up to that mirror of reality, we get a distorted reflection. Often the pain experienced in a crisis depends on how big a gap looms between what is real and what we wished would be.

Marsh's heart attack changed my image of who my husband really is. I had never given much conscious thought to his mortality. In the life-threatening crisis that brought Marsh to a bed in the coronary care unit, I saw what I had not noticed or thought about until then. Marsh is mortal. That means he will die. Maybe not now, but he won't live forever.

That thought came as a great surprise! I knew that I would die; that realization had come with my mother's death ten years earlier. But I had never applied that to Marsh. My image was of an invincible man. Not only was he physically strong and active, his energy for life had always seemed so unfaltering.

If I thought far enough into the future, to our eighties or nineties, I could imagine us aged and dying. But the day my image was shattered I was only forty-three.

Marsh was my first love. I "fell for him" when we were in high school. My image of him then was of a handsome, blue-eyed blond with an athlete's body, a scholar's mind, an intensity for life, and a powerful moral drive. Had I never looked at him again? Why hadn't I seen the twenty-three years of changes?

The man I saw looking out at me from the tubes, wires, and machinery in the cardiac care unit that night was a half-bald, gray-faced, middle-aged man. Where had my adolescent hero gone? Who was this sick and aging man, his blue eyes flecked with fear and disbelief?

Why had I never noticed time passing? Why had I never brought the image of my mate up to date? My percep-

tion of him was unconnected to the real world with its unrelenting passage of time.

As painful as it was to look time in the face, there was no way to avoid it. Little by little, reminded by my own graying hair and the lines in my face, I began to integrate my image of us, making it more accurate and realistically current. We are no longer teenage lovers, but our lives aren't over by any means. Now my image of us as vital human beings is enriched with the maturity and wisdom that comes with experience.

The pain of hanging on to something that you ought to let go of, or yearning for something that is already gone, can be eased. The cardiac crisis is one of those situations where you must look at your life's old "picture album." Nostalgia is to be expected. And reminiscences about the past can stimulate good memories and intimacy. But ultimately, your images may need an overhaul. Don't burn the album; see it clearly and then look at today's picture.

The images you construct can't keep you safe from pain. Janet, an adult cardiac daughter, experienced the pain of losing her childhood image of her father. To Janet, Dad was powerful and strong, a man who would always be there to protect her. The reality of his heart disease forced her to confront her outdated image of him. She witnessed her forceful father, now weak and dependent, requiring a nurse's help to urinate. The new reality required that Janet grieve, and gave her the opportunity to build an updated image of her dad.

The power of one person's images can influence another's. Edy, an earnest woman in her late thirties, relates, sadly, that her husband, Jake, has been calling himself "damaged goods" ever since his heart attack. He is so ashamed that he even suggested that Edy divorce him. Jake's image of himself has so strained their relationship that whenever Edy does anything for him, he accuses her of acting out of pity.

Both Jake and Edy are suffering because Jake has such a limited image of himself. Edy feels helpless, unable to convince Jake that her caring comes from love, and that she doesn't see him as "damaged." Only Jake can transform his image. If he doesn't, it will color his actions, diminish his self-esteem, and may even destroy his relationship with Edy.

In addition to personal images, there are cultural images to cope with. Cultural images influence us because large numbers of people accept them. For example, the great numbers of male cardiac bypass patients help establish an image of acceptance and normalcy. In some cardiac rehabilitation programs the bravado engendered by the cardiac camaraderie even suggests celebrity status. "Zipper chests" are recognized as a badge of courage, and cases are compared and discussed. Conversely, women having the same surgery suffer with a negative image of disfigurement and isolation. Women lack the "locker-room" opportunity for repartee, and are neither prepared nor given support. No one admires their scars or offers suggestions as simple as a front-closing bra, easier to negotiate after bypass surgery.

In general, it doesn't dawn on us to question the accuracy or virtue of cultural images. Some are correct reflections of reality, while others are distorted. It is crucial to question such popular misconceptions and images as that heart disease is a disease of old age, that heart disease only affects men, that heart disease is caused by high stress, that heart disease means the end of normal life - including exercise and all strenuous physical and sexual activity.

Brad, a cardiac spouse in his late fifties, told me how his and Polly's lives were limited by Polly's inaccurate image of herself. Brad first met Polly at a square dance. Although most of their interests were very different, they continued to square dance several times a month over the thirty-five years of their marriage. When Polly had a heart attack, she announced that her square dancing days were over.

Within a few months, Polly's physician gave her the go-ahead to resume her activities, including dancing, but she was too afraid to consider it. She encouraged Brad to go, but refused to accompany him to the dances, so Brad stayed home.

Square dancing became something that they couldn't talk about. She felt guilty that she had made him give up dancing, and he felt guilty wanting her to go. I asked them to share their worst fear. They both agreed it was that Polly would suffer another heart attack in the middle of a dance.

Once they had confronted their most terrifying image, their fear lost some of its power. They decided to go to the next weekend dance. Brad reported how excited and scared they were. Brad danced the entire evening. Polly alternated between dancing and sitting out. They went home early, and exhausted. But they had a wonderful time, reminiscing about the night they first met, discovering how happy they were to still have each other and dance, too.

Your own self-image can limit or free you. Start now to *redefine* and *update* your images of yourself and your mate. Bring your images up to date; letting go of the past allows you to live more fully in the present.

Updating Your Images

The nature of your reality is forever different because of the cardiac crisis. Acknowledging that the images you relied on are now shattered leaves you confused. The old image no longer fits, but you have yet to create a new one. You may understand intellectually that the image you had was inaccurate, but now what? What can you believe in? Where will you find new images that reflect reality more accurately? How can you create images for your new attitudes and actions?

Mending your broken images requires a courageous look; a clear assessment of the accuracy of your images as compared to an objective reality; the strength to let go of the inaccurate, outdated, or self-destructive; and a conscious effort to replace the old images with newer, healthier, more appropriate ones.

Here is a Heartmates® exercise designed to help you examine the images that presently motivate or direct your life. Use each set of questions as a guide. Respond with both your head and your heart. Don't be concerned about writing full sentences, making sense, or being logical. Use these questions to explore your images as fully as you can.

HEARTMATES® GUIDE FOR EXAMINING IMAGES

1. **What do you recall about first visiting your mate in the hospital?** See your mate and the coronary care unit as a still photo; then add sounds, smells, and movement to your image. What nonverbal message did you receive about your spouse's condition? In your mind's eye, see yourself then. What were you feeling, thinking, doing? Describe your communication, feelings, level of intimacy with your mate.

2. **Create an image of your mate's physical heart.**

As much as you can, visualize the actual damage as well as its symbolic meaning. Then see the healing that has occurred. How is your mate's physical and emotional heart different now from before the onset of heart disease? Based on your image, how do you envision the long-term quality of your mate's life? Imagine yourself five years, ten years, and twenty years into the future. What effects has your mate's heart disease had on your life? How do you expect the picture will continue to change?

3. **What image of home and family do you have from the period of active recovery?** What concerns did you have then about caring for your mate, your family, yourself? See in your mind's eye the network of communication and feelings that connected your family then. How was the family different during recovery from the way it was before the cardiac crisis? What is your image of your family now? As you see your family at present, note what issues your family is dealing with and what is going well for all of you.

4. **Look into a mirror of your past.** Who were you before your mate's heart crisis? What was important to you? What was your relationship with your mate like? How was your daily life organized? What were your priorities? How did you define your purpose for living? Gather this past image of you and set it aside.

5. **Stand in front of the same mirror right now. Who are you today?** What do you know about your strengths and limitations? How do you feel about yourself now? What is important to you today? What is your relationship with your mate like? How do you organize your daily life? What are your priorities? What is your purpose for living? Gather this present image of you and put it alongside your past image.

6. **Step back far enough so you can see both images in the mirror.** Visualize how being a cardiac spouse has changed you. What have you learned? How have you weathered the changes? How would you assess your acceptance of what's happened to you? Have you forgiven your mate, yourself? Are you taking care of your most important needs? Are you continuing to mourn your losses and heal your wounds?

Purposeful examination of our images allows us to update them continually as time passes and conditions change. One of the advantages of taking stock and comparing past and present images is that you can appreciate new qualities you've developed in yourself as a response to the cardiac crisis. Claire, who had always described herself as someone "with no head for figures," took over the family finances when her husband, Tim, was hospitalized because of a heart attack. Tim had always paid the bills, balanced the family checkbook, and made all the crucial financial decisions. Claire, busy with her weaving and other crafts, was satisfied to let Tim handle that aspect of their life; she wasn't interested and believed she was incompetent with numbers.

After four months of being the family banker, Claire confessed that she enjoyed keeping the books. She discovered that the more she worked with figures, the more her confidence grew. Tim even called her a "crack book-keeper." Claire occasionally still characterized herself in the old way, but when she told Tim, he just laughed. He reminded her of all the years she had never even subtracted her checks in the checkbook.

Recognizing your outdated images will help you disengage yourself from them. If you can catch yourself falling back on old images, you can learn to stop. Your mate may be willing to keep an eye out for behavior akin to your old images, to point out when you've limited yourself. Then you can consciously replace the old image with a new one that is more realistic and up to date.

What do you want your new images to be? What qualities do you want to develop? Some qualities a cardiac spouse could use are clarity, wisdom, love, strength, gratitude, humor, and forgiveness. Write the quality you desire most in large letters on a three-by-five-inch card. Colored pens or markers will permit you to choose the right color or your favorite color for the quality. Feel free to add a design that fits the quality you've chosen. Place the card where you will see it often, where it will attract your attention. The refrigerator door and the mirror above my bathroom sink are my favorite places. Look at the word each day to keep the image active in your mind, even when you aren't paying conscious attention. Visualize how you can express the quality in your daily life. When you stop noticing the card, move it to your bedside, or make a new, different colored card with different shaped letters to attract your attention. Keep that reminder in view.

SOME IDEAS TO REMEMBER ABOUT IMAGES

- Everyone has images.
- People experience their images differently: some people summon visual pictures, others sense their images.
- People respond to images as if they were reality.
- Images influence understanding, attitudes, and actions.
- Images can affect physical and emotional health.
- Creating new images requires conscious effort.
- Lost images need to be mourned.

- Defining yourself by an outdated image limits who you are and what you can do.
- Update your images and free yourself.

Forgiveness

The final step in the healing process is forgiveness. Mentally chastising yourself for your feelings clogs the process and impedes healing. Once you can understand and accept what has happened, you can be compassionate and forgiving of yourself.

One cardiac spouse, Betsy, has spent most of her time since Jeff's surgery berating herself for being angry. Even though she "knew" she should be grateful for Jeff's recovery, she couldn't stop feeling sorry for herself. The more she tried to be solicitous, covering her anger and pretending to be concerned only about Jeff, the more resentful she became. She was hurt that no one recognized or appreciated her pain despite the fact that she kept it to herself.

When Betsy was able to recognize that she was responsible for keeping herself isolated, the process of forgiveness began. As Betsy was able to release her feelings, she came to understand that she, too, had been wounded. Being gentle and forgiving toward herself also set the stage for her to be able to forgive Jeff.

When you get a sense of your mate's and your own mortality, your life comes into sharp focus. Forgiveness is motivated by the human longing for reconciliation. When there are fractures in relationships and unaccepted grievances, an attitude open to reconciliation can aid healing. The impulse, given the acknowledgment of mortality, is to "finish business" and clean up relationships.

Forgiveness usually demands a transformation in

attitude. Reluctance to give up a grievance may be the result of pride, stubbornness, or fear of rejection. If you are willing to humbly consider hurtful acts you have committed, apologize and make amends, you're already making a new start. The anxiety of strained relationships and wounded psyches is ameliorated by making restitution, which leads to forgiveness, a step on the journey to inner peace.

The cardiac patient and the cardiac spouse need to forgive the imperfection implied by heart disease. The illusion of perfection often crumbles with the onset of the cardiac crisis. Many heart patients experience deep anger at their bodies' betrayal; some consider divorce to punish themselves or to protect their spouses from having to live with "second-best."

Believing that you are worthwhile and that you deserve love just because you are human, not because you are perfect, is a major shift in thinking that requires real psychological effort. You need to end standing in judgment, accept and forgive your mate for his imperfections, including heart disease. Equally important, you need to accept and forgive yourself and God.

Sources of Support

No one can heal all alone. You need and deserve support and encouragement to get through your grief.

Physical Support. When you use so much of your vital and emotional energy to grieve, you need to pay special attention to your physical care. Take extra vitamins. Avoid physical excesses. Be sure you get the extra sleep you require. Use relaxing music rather than television as a sleep-inducer. Eat nutritious and good-tasting food. Include lots of fruits and vegetables in your diet. Drink six to eight glasses of water every day, and reduce or eliminate entirely caffeine and alcohol. Wear clothes that are comfortable, cozy, and warm. Take regular breaks from your routine, and stretch your muscles. Take a walk every day or stick to your regular fitness plan, but remember that this is not the time to start a strenuous, new exercise program. If possible, arrange to have regular therapeutic massage, because, "Grief tells the world that you are untouchable at the very moment when touch is the only contact that might reach you."14 See your physician for any physical symptoms of stress. If you question a specific activity, ask yourself, "Will this help me focus on my feelings?" This is not indulgent; it is essential for you to concentrate on your needs and keep your physical maintenance at a simple, stable level.

Emotional support. Here are some things you can do to support yourself emotionally. Listen to music that you find beautiful and harmonic. Treat yourself to soothing teas and favorite foods. Pamper yourself. Avoid isolation. Invite help from family and friends when you feel overwhelmed. Share your feelings with a trusted confidante. Stay away from places, people, and activities that are harsh or cold or overly demanding. Think of positive memories that evoke your feelings of pleasure and gratitude. Laugh aloud every day. If you have no friend or family member available, seek emotional support from a therapist or grief counselor. Seek out and participate in grief groups or recovery programs that energize optimism and empowerment. They may meet at your hospital, your church, or your local community center.

Spiritual Support. Many people find their spirits replenished in nature. Breathe deeply and inhale fresh air in your city park or along a country road to revitalize yourself. Nothing feels more nurturing than the warmth of the sun in the sky overhead and the security of the earth under your feet. Gardening has beneficial effects. Water is also healing to the spirit; take warm baths and frequent showers. Walk by your favorite lake or, if it's near, enjoy the ocean's powerful and repetitive sound and spray.

The cardiac crisis may have clarified how much of your energy and time has been given to others. Recognize that self-care requires more than attention to your body and feelings. Save time on a regular basis to be quiet, to give yourself the silence that can heal your wounded spirit.

It may be that the cardiac crisis has reawakened or deepened your religious connection. By accepting your limitations and turning to a greater source, your spirit will be nourished. Many people find that religious services and familiar rituals offer peace. Some may be comforted just sitting in a silent chapel. Others find profound value in prayer or meditation. Talk to your minister, priest, rabbi, or another spiritual leader. You know best what will help you. Make a commitment to support your spiritual self.

Turning Toward the Future

Time alone isn't enough to heal all wounds. But with the courage to face your pain and the willingness to update your images, active mourning does end! There are clues that you have grieved enough. You can mark your progress by the fact that your life has started to return to "normal." As you reorient yourself from the past into the present, more realistic images signal that you are healing.

One strong sign of recovery is commonly described as "a sense of release." A cardiac spouse realized her new freedom when whole days went by without her thinking about her spouse's heart condition or wishing for life as it used to be. Another spouse was delighted when he became aware that he was beginning to look ahead. He confidently made plane reservations for next winter's vacation with his mate.

Spontaneous and genuine interest in others is an important indication that the cardiac crisis is behind you. I remember with pleasure the cardiac spouse who declared enthusiastically that she was finally being released from the prison of her own pain. In the year since her husband's surgery, she had been so involved that she was barely able to tolerate conversation about anything other than her spouse's condition. Her world began to open like a flower as she anticipated spending meaningful time with friends and family again.

Another characteristic of healing is renewed energy. During the acute crisis and often in the long months of recovery, most of your vital energy was expended just to get through each day. Fatigue and exhaustion were common complaints. Now, gradually (or sometimes in a dramatic burst) you gain enough physical strength to do things that for months you've been unable to consider, let alone accomplish. You'll have renewed emotional energy; you may *want* to plant a garden, make plans with friends, and participate in leisure activities with or without your mate. You might pick up a stimulating novel or involve yourself in a new project.

That you can now make better judgments is another sign of your recovery. Of course, circumstances necessitated your making serious decisions long before this time, but the difference is qualitative. Recall how consuming and exhausting it felt to make decisions. Remember your confusion and frustration when you couldn't think things through? Now your ability to concentrate without undue effort has returned. Once again you can follow through fully and efficiently.

The return of regular eating habits and pre-crisis sleeping patterns, the easiest signs to measure, may be the last to occur. Things will change gradually, until you find that the present includes and integrates both the losses and lessons of the past and your newly crafted dreams for the future.

Lift up your eyes
Upon this day breaking for you.
Give birth again
To the dream.

Women, children, men,
Take it into the palms of your hands,
Mold it into the shape of your most
Private need. Sculpt it into
The image of your most public self.
Lift up your hearts
Each new hour holds new chances
For a new beginning.[15]

CHAPTER NOTES

1. The significance of grieving shattered dreams (the process I have described in this chapter as grieving the old image in order to update images, to reflect present reality and give hope for the future) was deepened again for me at a powerful professional workshop presented by Ted Bowman, MSW, only a few days before

this revised edition was due on my editor's desk. I refer you further to his self-published 1994 booklet, *Loss of Dreams: A Special Kind of Grief,* which can be ordered by writing him at 2111 Knapp Street, St. Paul, MN 55108, or by calling or faxing him at (612) 645-6058.

2. Hippocrates, *Precepts,* chapter 1, quoted in John Bartlett, *Familiar Quotations,* 13th ed. (Boston: Little, Brown & Co., 1955), p. 21.

3. See Norman Cousins' last book, *Head First: The Biology of Hope* (New York: E. P. Dutton, 1989).

4. Surviving the loss of their twenty-five year old son, who was struck by lightning, is a focus of Merton P. and A. Irene Strommen's book, *Five Cries of Grief* (San Francisco: HarperSanFrancisco, 1993). In it they differentiate five kinds of pain and grief, which is useful for understanding the pain experienced when we deal with any major change or loss.

5. See Stephanie Ericsson's *Companion Through The Darkness: Inner Dialogues on Grief* (New York: Harper-Collins, 1993), for the most eloquent and powerful writing on grief that I have ever read. How grateful I am that so far my grief is about loss far less devastating than hers, the loss of her spouse.

6. Addressing cardiac rehabilitation professionals in the state of Washington in 1992, I drove through the Yakima reservation and was fortunate to visit the museum of the Yakima Indian Nation, where their values and philosophy were displayed visually and in powerful words such as these. It was one of those special experiences when beauty and truth are present and so was I.

7. Elisabeth Kübler-Ross, *On Death and Dying* (New York: Macmillan, 1969).

8. See Kenneth R. Mitchell and Herbert Anderson, *All Our Losses/All Our Griefs* (Philadelphia: The Westminster Press, 1983), where they describe the symbolic,

intrapsychic losses as "the experience of losing an emotionally important image of oneself, losing the possibilities of 'what might have been,' abandonment of plans for a particular future, and the dying of a dream."

9. Amelia Earhart Putnam, *Courage*, quoted in John Bartlett, *Familiar Quotations*, 13th ed. (Boston: Little, Brown & Co., 1955), p. 981.

10. Joan Borysenko, Ph.D., *Fire In The Soul: A New Psychology of Spiritual Optimism* (New York: Warner Books, 1993), p. 16. She cites Shelley E. Taylor, whose research and writing is about people who have readjusted well after their lives have been disrupted by misfortune. Taylor isolates three coping strategies for optimal recovery: a search for meaning in the experience, an attempt to gain mastery over the event in particular and life in general, and a recouping of self-esteem after experiencing a loss.

11. William Shakespeare, *Macbeth*, Act IV, Scene iii, in *Twenty-three Plays and Sonnets*, ed. Thomas Marc Parrott (New York: Charles Scribner's Sons, 1953), p. 853.

12. Carl Simonton, S. Simonton, and J. Creighton, *Getting Well Again* (Los Angeles: Tarcher, 1978); and Jeanne Achterberg, Imagery in Healing (Boston: New Science Library, 1985).

13. Adapted from a broadcast on Minnesota Public Radio entitled "Positive Emotions and Health," on 8/9/85. Presented by Norman Cousins at St. John's Hospital and Medical Center, Santa Monica, California.

14. Stephanie Ericsson, *Companion Through The Darkness: Inner Dialogues on Grief* (New York: HarperCollins, 1993), p. 8.

15. Maya Angelou, *On The Pulse of Morning* (New York: Random House, 1993), from her poem written for and read at President William Jefferson Clinton's Inaugural Ceremony in Washington, D.C. on January 20, 1993.

Frogs Don't Turn Into Princes, But Men Become Heartmates

As a male cardiac spouse, *a man in crisis*, you have special needs. Cardiac spouses react like most people in a life-threatening emergency, but they have the unique experience of being in a crisis precipitated by someone else's illness. Coping with a mate's illness always presents difficult challenges, but when the heart patient is a woman and the cardiac spouse a man it is even more complicated.

As women in our culture have been trained to suppress their needs, men have been taught that it's manly to cover up feelings, to present a strong front. While some men may feel comfortable revealing feelings, most are inhibited or embarrassed about their sadness, fear, or anger. On the inside you may be devastated by your wife's illness; on the outside you remain stoic.

Men in our society have been educated to be breadwinners. Tradition from our cave-dwelling days describes men as providers, women as nurturers, and our patterns and life-styles remain similar today. Men learn early, from their mothers, to expect caretaking from women. It is rare in our culture for a man to assume the role of caretaker. But your wife has had a cardiac crisis and she needs you for caretaking and nurture as well as protection and financial security. How can you do and be everything for her as well as recover yourself from this sudden and unexpected life change?

Let's go one step at a time, and begin near the beginning of your cardiac story. You need to understand the issues, and accomplish the best possible recovery for you and your wife.

Out of the Loop - In The Hospital

Most cardiac events bring patients and their mates to the hospital. Once there, your wife embarks on her path toward a procedure or toward recovery. What are you to do? At the outset, you may feel like the water boy for the football team, standing on the sidelines hoping you'll be needed. Everyone but you has a job to do and appears busy and important. They may not even notice you standing at the nursing desk, looking lost. No one seeks you out to inform you or enlist your help.

Or you may find yourself suddenly thrown into the championship game as the quarterback. Without training or coaching you are responsible for calling the plays. Unless you have medical training, you are faced with a vocabulary of medical terms you can barely pronounce, let alone understand. The medical team's play-book is full of technical information difficult to decipher, which you may need to make life-and-death decisions on behalf of your mate. Worst of all, your wife, the person you count on as your offensive coordinator, is totally unavailable.

Your primary concern is for your mate's survival, but you also have to find your way in a new and strange environment. You'll be more effective for your recovery and hers if you take the time to find your way around. Explore the hospital - get to know the location of the family lounge, the telephone, the gift shop, the coffee shop, and the chapel - you will feel more secure and at ease.

Once you get your bearings, the next step is to figure out the inner workings of the system. You need to get familiar with the technical language as well as the schedule and routine on each shift. (The illustrations of heart disease in appendix A and the Glossary of medical terms near the end of this book can help you "crack the code"). There is nothing you can do to change the hectic tempo of your spouse's medical team, but you can work better within the system when you understand what's going on.

Next you face an issue that involves both your male strength and weakness. It's about getting the information you need, which requires asking questions of others. If it's hard for you to ask directions when you're lost driving your car, imagine how lost you are as your wife's heartmate. The direction you need and the questions you have on the road to recovery are very important. They may even have life-and-death implications.

But your nature has been not to ask, to go it alone. Male competency has depended on knowing, and men believe that it shows weakness to ask directions or information from others. You *should* be able to protect your wife and family without help from anyone. This is not a good time to rely on your "macho" image. The cardiac crisis is an extraordinary situation that requires you to summon all your courage, to ask questions, to get all the information you need to be the best possible protector of your wife and family. Lack of information, the unfamiliar hospital setting, difficult terminology, and the precarious nature of your mate's condition, contribute to your anxiety and helplessness. Voice your concerns and ask your questions to help you reduce your anxiety, frustration, and impatience.

How can you find an appropriate moment to discuss your concerns when the staff always seems so busy? You need to be as practical as they are. Set up a specific time with the nursing staff to get your questions answered. It's unlikely that you are going to change the doctors' schedules, but you can call your doctor's office to find out when he will be at the hospital or make a formal appointment to talk with him instead of anxiously waiting for his appearance every day.

Practical Suggestion #1: Phone the doctor's office to arrange a time to get your questions answered.

Tim reported his meeting with the specialist: "The doc told me my wife was not a candidate for bypass surgery. It felt as if he were an auto mechanic telling me my car couldn't be fixed. I should just take it home and run it until it won't run anymore." When others are insensitive, your situation can be more difficult. Your doctor may be highly respected for his expertise, but his bedside manner may leave lots to be desired. In most cases asking questions and looking for direction will help you maneuver more effectively and negotiate more ably for your wife and yourself.

Put your questions in writing to help you remember them and ensure your efficiency. Once you have compiled a list, decide who is the appropriate member of the medical team for each of your questions. Some concerns should be directed to your family doctor or the cardiologist. Others require the expertise of the nursing staff or a veteran cardiac spouse. Write down the answers to your list of questions; that way you can go over them again in detail. It is your need, your right, and your responsibility to have access to *all* the available data. Use the medical staff as a resource to help you find out what you, your spouse, and your family are battling, and how it will affect your lives.

Practical Suggestion #2: Buy a pocket-sized notebook and write down your questions and the answers.

Male cardiac spouses often perceive the hospital staff as a lifeline of support and care for their wives. What a relief not to bear the responsibility alone! But then you may also feel dependent on them. Then you may feel unsure about whether to express your opinions. You may doubt the value of your non-professional input, even fear that it will be misconstrued by staff as interference or doubt. But remember, *you are the most important source of information about the patient; you know your wife better than anyone else.* Sharing your knowledge can be crucial in planning the most appropriate recovery program for her, and most hospital staff members will respect your expertise and knowledge.

You also need to feel useful and needed during your wife's hospitalization. It looks as if the competent professional staff takes care of everything - what could you possibly accomplish? But you are needed; your wife needs you!

There are things you can do directly for her that she can't do for herself in the hospital. Moistening her dry lips, moving a sheet that's pulling on a tube, or readjusting a pillow: these small acts make her comfortable and express your caring. That's important for you and her. Functioning as a knowledgeable intermediary between your wife and the busy professional staff can make her hospital stay easier for everyone. Keeping her posted about the events of your daily life and those of close family members and friends will strengthen her commitment to recover. By communicating for your wife when she's unable to do it for herself, and by communicating with your wife to encourage her interest in getting well, you are making significant contributions to her recovery.

Practical Suggestion #3: Inform hospital staff about what your wife needs. Tell your wife about what's going on outside the hospital.

Your presence itself is significant to your wife because you are a symbol of stability and reality for her at a time of extreme confusion and vulnerability. As the bread-winner and the family protector your success depends on how well you solve problems. But caregiving is different; it's not about action or you taking the Mr. Fixit role. It's about *being and listening. You* may be more comfortable when you can arrange pillows and bring her a glass of water, but your wife needs you just to listen to her concerns. The support and love you offer by your willingness to be with your wife in the hospital and during rehabilitation at home is an important contribution to her recovery.

You need to take time daily to "withdraw into the cave of your mind,"[1] to reduce the added stress of not being able to solve all the problems of your wife's heart disease. Give yourself permission to get away: read your newspaper, watch your favorite TV show or sporting event, or take on your favorite tennis opponent. A challenge that is 180 degrees from your concerns about heart disease will renew your energy. Once you have released your tension, you can redirect your focus and give your wife the attention she needs.

Practical Suggestion #4: Withdraw regularly into

activities you find challenging or interesting to release tension and renew your energy.

Balancing the Two Sides of a Coin

Giving makes you feel strong and competent. But it's equally important to be able to receive. In the acute period of a cardiac crisis, every one's focus is understandably on the patient. However, you, too, are in crisis; you are physically and emotionally vulnerable. Your daily schedule has been disrupted, you are spending many hours at the hospital, you are deeply affected by your wife's illness, and you are trying to juggle her needs with all the other demands in your life.

Taking care of yourself may be a totally new concern. You may have depended on your wife to oversee this aspect of your life, but for now, she's not available. So you need to be responsible about arranging time to take care of yourself. Be sure you are getting enough rest, and that you are eating well. Take a walk at least once a day. Let your friends and relatives give to you. A warm meal delivered to your home, company in the waiting room or walking around the hospital grounds, a visit with your wife so that you aren't solely responsible, a card game to distract your mind; these offerings from loved ones let you take a break, get a much-needed "time out."

Many hospitals offer an educational program to provide rehabilitation information: about diet, exercise, risk factors, stress, and sexuality. These classes are to prepare the two of you for going home. Even if the focus of this education is about your wife's recovery needs, remember that *you* are in crisis, too. You can consider what's rehabilitation for your wife as good health maintenance for you. Think of these programs as a resource to help both of you change your life-styles to be more heart-healthy.

Practical Suggestion #5: Apply the hospital education program to your health. Eat regularly, get the sleep you need, do daily exercise.

Your powers of concentration, focus, and retention are reduced when you are in crisis. Seek information more than once if you forget or need details repeated. Use your notebook to write the answers as well as the questions you ask. This "team playbook" might be an ideal place to record things you can't remember: the name of the nurse in charge, the times that hospital shifts change, phone numbers of people you may need to contact. If you have the name of a nurse you trust, you can call her at the hospital with a question even after you've been home a while.

Practical Suggestion #6: Write down details; you may find them useful later.

Remember, the hospital experience is the beginning of a life-long process heralded by the cardiac crisis. Issues that begin here will follow you home. Ongoing contact with the medical community is a part of life with someone who has heart disease. A positive way to approach this is to develop a relationship with the hospital caregivers. Many hospitals sponsor clubs or programs for cardiac couples to meet regularly to discuss concerns: new medications, heart-healthy food plans, smoking cessation, and behavioral changes precipitated by the cardiac event are a few familiar program topics. Some programs include teaching about stress reduction, relaxation, and maintaining a positive attitude.

More people criticize their weaknesses than give themselves credit for how well they've handled a crisis. It's easier to focus on mistakes or second-guess decisions than to appreciate the positive qualities that enhance recovery. If you are going to cope successfully with the changes of heart disease, you need to appreciate what has happened to *you* and how you've responded. Look at yourself and your situation objectively. How have you met the challenge of your mate's life-threatening cardiac crisis? Take a hard look at reality, but don't sell yourself short. You may be used to getting appreciation from your wife, but her energy is now focused on *her* recovery.

Acknowledge and affirm your strengths. Take credit where credit is due. Encourage yourself to continue on the road to recovery. Cardiac spouses are awe inspiring in crisis. Just look: You have the *courage* to ask questions. Your *patience* lets you listen to your wife's concerns even when there are no solutions you can offer. You express *love* by being with her. Your *organizational skills* enable you to be responsible at work, at home, and at the hospital, too. Each cardiac spouse is unique and has his own qualities. Name yours, and give yourself the pat on the back you deserve.

Practical Suggestion #7: Look at your strengths and appreciate yourself every day.

When the Tables Are Turned

When your wife is discharged from the hospital, your hopes are high for her recovery. You leave nothing behind. Once home you unpack the cards, the gifts, and the plants she received, and you also bring home the relationship patterns that began with your wife's diagnosis. You find yourself in the position of caretaker. Without training or preparation, you are expected to have an instant aptitude for nursing, household maintenance, even child care. With the woman as the recovering patient and the man as the caretaking cardiac spouse, the traditional male and female roles have reversed.

Early in the cardiac crisis the basic elements of your life-style are the most noticeably affected. At a time when you especially need nourishment and rest, you are coping with new dietary requirements and disrupted sleep. And for the first time in your life, you may be totally responsible for meal preparation and grocery shopping. No aspect of your life is immune to this crisis. Your work schedule, leisure time, and social life have been interrupted and altered. Your primary relationship is also in transition. And your personal goals and dreams, beliefs and values, are undergoing change as a result of your mate's heart disease.

If you feel concerned by the change of roles and responsibilities in your family, you are not alone. Most men feel overwhelmed by the new demands thrust upon them. It's not unusual to hear a cardiac spouse say that just sitting at the hospital is difficult and that he wished he could express his caring in a more active way. Even the most devoted husband will feel pressured and inadequate with his wife's need for emotional support. Remember that your presence *is* a support.

Your first serious trip to the supermarket may make you think you've been abandoned on an alien planet. Even if the layout of the store is familiar, having to find items low in sodium and fat requires familiarity with the foreign language of food labeling. Surviving the supermarket is only the beginning. The next stop is the kitchen, where the utensils are arranged according to some indecipherable code. Finding the tools and making a meal for a heart patient is stressful for all cardiac spouses. It is especially challenging for men whose experience and expertise normally lead them to the workshop, not the kitchen.

Adopting a heart-healthy diet is the number one concern for many couples in the early stages of recovery. Before the cardiac crisis your responsibility for diet and food may have been to sit down at the table and push away when you were finished. Now, at least for a period of time, you are the leader in the task of reshaping the family's eating habits into a heart-healthy diet. Although a heart-healthy diet is not much different from the general trend toward nutritious eating, for the cardiac family it involves more than being fashionable or fit. It feels like a matter of life and death.

Directing your mate's diet, watching what she eats, counting fat grams and monitoring salt intake, is usually an attempt to maintain control in a situation that is overwhelming. Managing diet is practical and can be broken into moderate-sized steps, a blessing when everything is so complicated. There is no diet plan that will assure immortality, no one way to prepare food so that it's right for every family. During the transition to a heart-healthy diet, communication is every bit as important as cuisine. You and your wife need to talk about the many changes heart disease has brought to your household and negotiate how to cope with this ongoing adjustment in your lives.

Practical Suggestion #8: Plan together and agree on the dietary changes you want to make.

Practical Suggestion #9: Don't try to change everything at once. Lasting change is done in small steps. Celebrate your successes together.

Steve, known to his family and friends as the strong, silent type, described how he struggled to express his caring and love to his wife. He had never been effusive, and, like many men of his generation, he was uncomfortable articulating his feelings. Steve loved Jean dearly. After her heart attack, he showed his concern by doing all the household chores after his regular long hours at work. He was particularly proud of his vacuuming. Jean didn't appear to appreciate Steve's efforts or to realize that his cleaning was a way to say, "I love you." As soon as she was well enough, Jean resumed vacuuming and her other chores. Steve felt frustrated with Jean's perfectionism and afraid that she was pushing herself too fast. Mostly he felt useless and incompetent. Jean, needing to test her own fitness after her heart attack, did what she knew best: reclaimed her role by taking over her household tasks. Because the feminine role is to be the caretaker, Jean probably was uncomfortable being cared for, as well as guilty about Steve doing both of their jobs. She unknowingly failed to appreciate her heartmate, Steve, in her haste to recover.

Like all cardiac spouses Steve needed support and understanding. Asking for support is difficult for men in our culture. It's natural for men to be shy, ashamed, or unwilling, assuming that to ask for help implies weakness. Men generally believe they should be able to handle everything alone. If you are holding back but need help — whether it's a hand with the cooking, or a shoulder to cry on — go ahead, ask. In a cardiac crisis you need and deserve all the support you can get!

Practical Suggestion #10: Remind yourself every day that you are okay even if you need help or support; a cardiac crisis is an extraordinary, not an ordinary, time.

Since they did not talk about their thoughts or feelings, Jean had no way to see that Steve was expressing love for her by taking over her tasks, and Steve didn't understand that Jean was eager to resume her chores because she felt helpless stripped of her habitual roles and activities. Whether the differences between men and women are caused by hormones or homemaking doesn't matter. What's important is that men and women understand and appreciate their inherent or learned differences so that the differences don't distance them from one another.

With all our society's sophisticated technology, we don't communicate very differently from the way we did when we lived in caves. Too often we rely on single-syllable grunts rather than telling each other how we feel. How different Steve might have felt had Jean explained that she felt uncomfortable, helpless, and guilty that Steve was taking care of her. Her role was to take care of their nest, and she was ashamed to see him vacuuming and cooking. And how differently Jean might have reacted had she known that she had taken away Steve's ability to *do* for her, and that he no longer felt useful or needed.

Practical Suggestion #11: Recognize ways that you and your wife are different. Remember those differences are inherent, not an indictment of you or her.

When you are anxious, it can be comforting to do things in habitual ways. A woman patient explained to her friend who had come over to help, "Jim tried to help me by doing the laundry, but I saved these loads for you. He washes it all together, he fills the machine too full, and he drys everything in the dryer. Men just don't understand about the laundry." You can't know exactly how your wife feels, and she can't completely understand how her illness has affected you. The best you can hope for is to be tolerant and appreciative of your differences. Remember that the crisis has been difficult for both of you.

In order to provide your wife with the attention and support she needs, it is essential for you to maintain your own health and well-being. Caring for her, you may assign your own needs, for sleep, healthy eating, and regular exercise, too low a priority. Interrupted or fitful sleep is a natural reaction to stress. Once the initial numbness and shock wear off, you still remain tense and on guard. Many cardiac spouses report awakening suddenly in the middle of the night and listening to make sure she's still breathing; then it's hard to fall back to sleep. That's par for the course. If your whole life could change in a cardiac second, it might happen again at any time. You are responding to the continuing threat of danger. The initial crisis has passed, yet you find it difficult to relax and sometimes to sleep.

Recovering cardiac patients often sleep fitfully, too, and need naps during the day. This change may be temporary, caused by the new medications and the trauma of a heart attack or cardiac procedure. Irregular sleep or changes in your mate's sleeping patterns aren't necessarily danger signals or something for you to be concerned about. Still, it may take months before you sleep peacefully again.

The old pattern of your wife paying attention to you and your needs disappeared when heart disease became a part of your reality. You wonder how long all her energy will be used on herself, her disease, her symptoms, her recovery. You have been left to fend for yourself without a word of explanation or a promise that the tables will turn again. Almost as quickly as you think such thoughts, you feel guilty and selfish: She might have been lost to me forever; how can I think of myself? But the thoughts don't go away, and they *are* normal. And paradoxically, many female patients are unable to accept or appreciate being taken care of; the meaning of their lives was defined by being the caretaker before heart disease, and they can't let go. These women respond to their mates' caring with irritability, anger, impatience, and criticism.

Just as her body struggles to adjust to her new diet and medications, your mind may keep you awake as it grapples with the many-leveled changes in your lives.

Shifting Gears

One of the biggest concerns you may wrestle with is in the arena of work. Whether your wife retires, changes vocation, or returns to her old job, your input is a valuable part of the decision-making process. You may hesitate to express your opinion because you don't want to add stress to an already difficult situation. But the stress already exists. Your questions and concerns are probably similar to your wife's.

Coping with work changes can be extremely stressful for both of you. There is no one right answer for any cardiac couple, except to keep the lines of communication open. Avoiding issues won't make them disappear. Ignoring such a sensitive topic may become a bigger problem than confronting it head on. Even if your wife's income was a fraction of yours, it may have meant more to her than the money itself. She may be grieving other lost satisfactions of work as well: what will her future provide to replace the fulfillment of doing something worthwhile? And not having money she earned may cause her to feel too dependent for her own comfort. Seek professional counsel if you and your wife can't talk about work-related issues.

Although you may have been the primary bread-winner in your family, the delay of your wife's return to work, or her early retirement, may add pressure to your lives during the recovery period and beyond. You may wonder how you will ever again be able to afford your life-style. You worry about medical bills piling up. You fear you'll be unable to support your children as they leave the nest and head for technical school or college. The pre-cardiac plans you shared for early retirement may be lost. The reality of heart disease may mean that you have to postpone your retirement because your wife may need to reduce her work. The pressure to be the sole provider for your family may also be directly at odds with what you want to do most since the onset of heart disease - spend more time with your wife.

It is very important that you and your wife take the time to talk about your feelings and make decisions together about the changes in your economic plan, as well as the ways the two of you choose to spend your leisure time. Even if your feelings on these subjects aren't similar, two heads are better than one as you seek creative ways to adjust to your new life-style and time constraints.

Practical Suggestion #12: Talk to your wife about your concerns about work and money issues.

Down Shifting

Obviously, your social and leisure activities have been affected by the cardiac life-style. What before seemed a simple decision - whether to go to a movie or play doubles tennis - becomes a major issue in adjusting to a heart-healthy life. You want to protect your wife's health, but at the same time maintain your friendships and social interests.

You may question her motivation, feel impatient, or even harbor resentment that she isn't improving more quickly. Men ask, "Why is she so tired? Why is she still depressed? Why isn't she feeling better by now?" You may need to alter your expectations during recovery. The cardiac patient needs time and psychological space to integrate the many changes resulting from heart disease. Pete planned a trip to Disney World for his recovering wife, their children, and grandchildren, thinking that such a vacation would bring Mattie's spirits up. When we discussed the normal pattern of Mattie's recovering in fits and starts, some days feeling down, wanting only to sit at home, and other days having more energy, Pete understood that it was *his* anxiety about Mattie's depression that was the impetus for what would be a strenuous trip for all of them. To Mattie's relief, Pete canceled the reservations and dealt with their grandchildren's disappointment. Crossing the bridge from active recovering to full recovery takes time, effort, and patience.

There isn't anything you can do to speed up the recovery process. However there are ways to adapt to it. During this period, you may ask your friends to be more flexible in accommodating your needs. Hopefully they will be understanding and tolerant of the situation. A rigorous night at the bowling alley may occasionally be replaced by a quiet evening watching movies on the VCR and munching salt-free popcorn; other times you may go to the bowling alley and leave your wife with a good book.

As the weeks go by and your wife's physical recovery moves forward, you may wonder when it's appropriate to return to your hobbies, activities, meetings, and friendships. At what point is it okay to resume your weekly golf game, poker night with the guys, or the monthly Lions meeting? You may think that the seriousness of heart disease precludes recreation and fun. Some cardiac spouses are afraid of criticism, worrying that being seen in public "having a good time," when a spouse has suffered a heart attack, implies that they are insensitive, uncaring, or selfish. Others just don't feel the old enthusiasm for projects that were important before all this began. You need to wean yourself gradually from habits that began as caretaking at the hospital when your wife was weak, vulnerable, perhaps in pain. Leave your wife alone for a short time at first, to grocery shop, meet a friend for breakfast, or go out for a run.

Once you return to work, your days will feel more normal. But there is more to life than work. As the weeks become months, planning your time apart is a way to respect your individuality and your wife's. She needs to reclaim activities, tasks, and roles that you took over when she couldn't do them for herself.

The choice about when you resume activities is an individual matter. It's very important to be involved in something besides work and caring for your recovering mate. Before your wife's cardiac event, you took the structure of your life for granted; returning to that order will increase your sense of control and safety. Whether you work in the yard, rearrange your tool room, go fishing or golfing, making time for *yourself* every day will help you heal. The guilt that attends wanting to "do your own thing" must be overcome! Maintaining interests in the broad areas of your life is essential for your recovery and will be paramount in restoring a healthy balance in your relationship.

Practical Suggestion #13: Say "no" to guilt. Your healing depends on you resuming activities that are nurturing to you.

Practical Suggestion #14: Talk together every week to plan time apart from each other; renegotiate as recovery unfolds.

The Emotional Poker Game

During the initial phases of the cardiac crisis, it is normal for you to feel numb and shaky, to have trouble concentrating, and difficulty staying focused on conversations with friends and relatives. These are typical reactions. Throughout the earliest phase of the cardiac crisis, it is wise to limit yourself to facing only those tasks and decisions that absolutely cannot wait.

As your numbness wears off, you will become aware of your fear. The most compelling of your terrors is that you'll lose your mate, and in the acute crisis even small things feel disproportionately threatening. Your fears may be expressed in various ways, including loss of appetite, trembling, shallow breathing, edginess, or insomnia. Fear paralyzes some people, makes others withdrawn, causes still others to become jittery or restless, irritable or angry. Everyone has a hard time coping with the unknown! Learning to live with uncertainty is the greatest challenge of the heartmate. Knowing that your wife is in competent professional hands may reduce your fear, but until your wife is home and recovering well for more than a few weeks, it's normal for your fear to surface.

The first six months of recovery is a particularly difficult period for you to adjust to, as an individual and as a couple. While there is much to be thankful for, transition is ever-present - your life continues to change and you're dealt uncertainty on a regular basis. The changes may be both obvious and subtle. At the onset of the cardiac crisis, there were major ruptures in your relationship. You were physically separated from each other with one in the hospital, the other at home. Limited hospital visits, protecting your wife from stress, and disguising your feelings of fear and anxiety caused a breakdown in communication.

Some couples carry that protective emotional distance into recovery and beyond. Although you may not be aware of it, it takes a lot of energy to keep your poker face on, to hide your feelings from your wife. In the long run, your energy is depleted, and it's easier to fold than to pursue your dealt hand and heal your relationship.[2] Setting up a pattern that inhibits intimacy and honesty will help neither of you heal.

Practical Suggestion #15: Take three minutes for sharing every day. Tell your wife one thing you are feeling and ask her to share one feeling with you. No solutions or responses are required of either of you. Just listen!

It is natural to push away unwanted feelings during the height of the emergency. Although she may not say anything either, your wife is probably experiencing feelings similar to yours. She is coping with the physical adjustments to heart disease, and with the emotional effects as well. Both of you need permission to have, not hide, *all* the feelings you are feeling, including the negative ones.

First, you must recognize what your feelings are. The royal flush of the emotional poker hand for cardiac spouses is dealt by the king of darkness. . . fear. The unexpected threat of losing the person most precious to you causes deep fear and anxiety. These emotions don't just go away, even when full recovery is the real outcome of a cardiac event. We live in an instant age, and we take for granted a speed unheard of in earlier times: jet travel, thirty-second bytes, faxes. So it's not surprising that we expect ourselves to heal from our mate's cardiac crisis at the speed of light. Full recovery does not mean than you have no more fear. Most people will continue to experience fear, though diminished with time, for years. Your body learned to respond to the crisis with anxiety reactions, and continues to respond, for a long time unable to differentiate between a cough and a cardiac arrest.

Almost ten years after Marsh's heart attacks and bypass surgery, I was surprised by how close to the surface was my fear. It was a beautiful August Saturday afternoon, and Marsh was out on the golf course. I had just come in from weeding my garden when the phone rang. Answering it, I heard an unfamiliar voice, "Mrs. Levin?" "Yes," I responded. I could already feel anxiety churning deep inside.

"This is Mrs. J___ from the golf course," she said. I knew my worst fantasy was about to come true. "Yes," I said, trying to hurry her telling me the dreadful news. The uncertainty was so painful and I was sure that I had lost my mate. She continued, "We're wondering if you and your husband would like to join our bowling league this fall?"

I had thought I was totally recovered from such fear; after all, it had been years. But the wound of the heartmate scars over and remains beneath the surface.

Anxiety may be expressed as a physical symptom in the body (sleeplessness, headaches, lack of appetite, tense and aching muscles) and an overwhelming feeling of helplessness. Many men try to reduce their anxiety by keeping busy, doing something to feel more in control. There are useful things to do that can help to relieve your anxiety and simultaneously protect your spouse.

Practical Suggestion #16: Visit your local fire

station. Familiarize the medics with where you live. They may be able to code your address screen on the 911 program to indicate that your wife is a heart patient.

The first step in dealing with anxiety is admitting to yourself that you are afraid. For most, the fear is about losing your wife. Once recognized, you can use logic. Ask yourself about the evidence for your anxiety, and then act appropriately. What is the *real* danger in this situation? Are there other symptoms beyond the cough you hear? What is your wife's assessment of the situation? An exception is the chronic anxiety when your wife's situation *is* severe and increasingly debilitating, as in congestive heart failure.

Another emotion hidden behind your poker face is anger. Although no feeling is logical, you may have a variety of reasons for your anger. You may be angry at the hospital professional staff or at your family for failing to recognize *your* needs. You may be angry at something as vague and abstract as your wife's heredity or genes. You may feel angry about how your life has changed, and about the additional responsibility you have taken on to be both provider and caretaker. If you're used to relying on your wife to meet many of your emotional needs, you may be angry about her neglect. It is important to recognize your feelings of anger - it is also useful to monitor your expression of feelings. *Expressing anger[3] at your wife will not endanger her health.* There are many appropriate ways to express anger safely; direct communication of it is the most effective.

Practical Suggestion #17: Tell your wife you're angry and frustrated. Find safe, physical outlets for your anger: hit any kind of ball as hard as you can; run or

swim. Use the angry energy to keep you strong and firm.

The energy sapped by unexpressed anger may leave you feeling sad and alone. We take our lives for granted until something threatens our security; then we experience enormous feelings of loss. *It is absolutely normal for you to feel depressed and disappointed.* As you yearn for things past, for your secure, pre-cardiac life, you are letting yourself grieve what you've lost. Our society honors those who make quick decisions and avoid pain. But each of us is unique, and we each grieve at our own pace. You may be tempted to minimize or deny your own sadness on the pretense of sacrifice. Feeling bad is not a sign of weakness, craziness, or failure. Give yourself the time *you* need to recover from the emotional trauma of the cardiac event and all the changes that have occurred since, just as you are tolerant about the time your wife needs to recover from the physical trauma she has been through.

Guilt is another key card in the deck of the cardiac spouse's feelings. Many men feel guilty about their mates' heart disease. They think they should have been able to prevent it, and feel guilty that they didn't. Even as our culture moves toward gender equality, we hold on to the belief that good men are successful providers and protectors. You need to maintain perspective on the situation. There is no way that you could have protected your wife from suffering a cardiac event. Wiring an alarm system or installing special door and window locks may protect against intruders, but you have no special skills to protect your wife from heart disease. Paradoxically, many men feel guilty when they want their wives to reestablish their caretaking responsibilities and to resume sexual relations, to be well again. Others feel guilt for taking her and her health for granted. And yet others experience guilt when they want to return to their well life activities.

Men may also feel guilty about being queasy or turned off seeing their wife's incision or scar after open heart surgery. Men's scars are actually considered handsome by many in our culture, or at least scars symbolize bravery. But not so for women, whose bodies are supposed to be perfect. Logically men can tell themselves not to feel the way they do, that the chest scar from open heart surgery is not as disfiguring as many others; but logic doesn't change what may actually be a physical reaction of nausea. Hiding disgust and the guilt that comes with it behind a poker face will not change how you feel; expressing it may help to minimize the feeling. Share your feelings with a friend.

Practical Suggestion #18: Acknowledge your guilty feelings. If your guilt will be burdensome to your wife, share with a friend, or write your feelings in a private place.

Male Bonding - The Need for Camaraderie

Sometimes it is important to enlist a friend, one willing to listen to your feelings without making judgments. Other times solitude is exactly what you need to sort through your varied feelings and whirling thoughts. Working through a crisis is a highly personal experience, but too much isolation is detrimental to recovery. If you hold everything tight to your chest and never show your hand, your healing will only be partial. But sharing needs to be timely, confidential, and respected by your confidant.

Unfortunately, when you're ready to talk, to share deep feelings with another, there may not be someone around willing to listen. Friends and family are most available to help during the early days of your crisis, but they may need prompting after weeks have passed and your wife has returned home. It's not easy to ask for support, especially if it isn't offered directly. Try to send clear messages about your needs to your family and friends and take advantage of offers for meals, child care, or even financial aid if you need assistance.

Practical Suggestion #19: Don't say, "No, no, that's okay, I'm doing fine." Learn to use the phrase: "Yes, thank you," when someone offers you help.

While family and friends are those who know you best and longest, they don't have first-hand knowledge about what you've experienced. There is great comfort in hanging out with a group of guys who have lots in common. Charlie called Fred, his old home-town pal, a couple of months after Joan's heart attack and subsequent procedure. He was relieved to hear Fred's voice and his concern. Fred was coming to the city and thought they should get together. Charlie agreed, looking forward to some time away from Joan, with a friend he could just be himself with. When they met, Charlie told Fred how scared he had been, and how frustrated and guilty he felt because Joan's recovery was taking longer than Charlie had expected. He felt good laying everything on the table and having Fred value how strong he'd been when Joan needed him. They decided to get together regularly when Fred came to the city on business, and Charlie returned home re-energized.

Reaching out to others who have lived through similar cardiac experiences can help you and them heal. Attend educational and support programs at your local hospital, both with your spouse and by yourself. The experience of telling your story to someone else and releasing the weight of your worries is an essential step in your recovery.

The toughest part of your recovery may be realizing and accepting that you can't do everything. In extraordinary circumstances, like a cardiac crisis, the pattern that men have to be strong, silent, and handle everything alone needs to be temporarily set aside. In order to recover, you need to reach out to family and friends and ask for help.

Taking Care of Business

A question I asked male cardiac spouses in this revision's questionnaire was: What was the hardest thing for you when she first came home from the hospital? Here are some typical answers. "Trying to keep her from working too hard." "Preventing her from doing work around the house." "Making sure she took her medication on time required me to keep a strict schedule." "Keeping her from moving ahead too fast (in my judgment)." "Not letting her do too much." Although I knew that most female cardiac spouses tend to be overly protective of their husbands, I was surprised to hear echoes of the very same attitude from male spouses. Notice how responsible each sounds - judging, taking responsibility for, keeping her, preventing her, not letting her.

What causes your caring to cross the line and become caretaking? It's that uncomfortable feeling of helplessness. Because you can't change the fact that your wife has heart disease, you compensate by taking charge. The power struggles that result from spouses overprotecting patients are legendary among cardiac couples. The more you try to get her to do less, the more she does.

Heart patients can be frightened when their mates pressure them to do less. Does my husband know something the doctor didn't tell me? Am I worse than I thought?

Husbands trying to control the uncontrollable come to believe their wife's recovery is in their hands. *It's not. You neither caused her heart disease, nor do you have the power to cure it.* But believing otherwise can backfire. The more you feel responsible for her, the more she resists. The more she resists, the more you feel unappreciated for the solutions you're suggesting. What she needs is to know that you love her.

Practical Suggestion #20: Show your strength and power by listening to your wife without telling her what to do or how to do it. Give her a hug and tell her you love her.

What you've taken on is doomed to failure: not because of your incompetence, but because you can't live *her* life, do *her* recovery, or keep *her* alive. No matter how much you love her, you cannot take basic responsibility for her. And the more your energy is focused on her recovery, the less attention you pay to your own.

Getting in Touch Again

Many people think of intimacy in its most limited definition, having sex. But intimacy, an essential component of recovery, needs to be understood more broadly. In his novel, *A Soldier of the Great War*, Mark Helprin poignantly expresses the human dilemma of love and mortality:

"...I see that the most beautiful thing between a man

and a woman is not the consummation of their love, but, simply, their regard for one another."

"That may be so, but you probably can't know it until you're condemned to die."

"You're always condemned to die. It's just a matter of timing."[4]

Being in recovery together can be an opportunity to express your regard for each other. Many couples find their awareness heightened, their hearts expanded, by heart disease. What you may have taken for granted before heart disease is now experienced as precious. You may come to appreciate each other more and find new ways to express your love.

One thing you both need now is to give and receive physical comfort. Holding hands and walking arm in arm, hugging and kissing, cuddling and spooning, are warm ways to get back "in touch" with your partner again. Be sure not to change pre-cardiac crisis sleeping arrangements. The physical separation when she was in the hospital was hard on both of you; stay sleeping in your bed together. Each knowing that the other is there, and reaching out to touch each other, is comforting.

Middle-aged and older couples have neither the physical energy nor the emotional desire to make love the way they did in their twenties and thirties. That may be hard to admit in our culture, which idolizes and idealizes youth and its beauty. But what we see on television and at the movies is not real life. Beauty and love belong to everyone if we dare to see it and live it. What is special is *you and your wife* being together the way you really are. Physical caring is expressed throughout life and all over the world in as many different ways as there are people. Your renewed discovery of each other, your soft, quiet embrace, may mean more to each of you than you ever imagined.

Although you've been through the sexual revolution of the sixties, you were taught even earlier that sex was private, so it's difficult to talk about. Here, then, is an opportunity for you to be courageous. Expanding your intimacy includes telling each other how you feel. Tell your wife how glad you are that she has survived the cardiac crisis, how lonely it was without her, how wonderful it is to hold her in bed again, that you miss being close to her, that you love her. Talking about sex begins with small steps. Tell her what *you* want and need, and ask her how she feels, and what she wants and needs.

Software and Hard Drive

It is unusual for women to have heart disease prior to menopause. Thus the average age of male heartmates is older than their female counterparts. Your level of activity as well as your attitudes about sex are subject to your age and to your being male.

Male cardiac spouses do have specific questions and expectations about sex. Part of your journey through the recovery period is trying to understand how sex fits into the "new normal" that is life with a mate who has heart disease. The most common questions include: Will having sex hurt her? Will sex risk her life? Why is she so disinterested in sex, and me? Does she still care about me? Will her attitude change as time goes on? How much is she affected by heart disease and how much by the normal aging process?

Let's begin with the physical aspects. The medical literature indicates that by six weeks after a cardiac event most heart patients can resume their normal activities, including sex. It takes about that long for the heart to heal after a heart attack, and perhaps slightly longer for women's breastbones and incisions to heal after open-heart surgery. After a balloon angioplasty or a cath procedure, if your wife has not had a heart attack, the restrictions about physical activity, including sex, are to wait twenty-four hours so that the puncture site has safely closed.[5] Because most studies have focused on male subjects, less is known about women's recovery, but what is clear is that physical recovery is unique to every individual.

When we look at the emotional dimension of a cardiac event and the return to sexuality, the picture gets more complicated. Some women are not interested in sex because they are depressed. *Depression is normal for cardiac spouses and patients* off and on for as much as a year after a cardiac event. People who are depressed lack energy and are disinterested in all kinds of activities that were normal for them before the crisis, including sex. Some men respond to emotional crisis with physical impotence. If that happens to you and more than a few weeks pass, talk with your doctor about it. Talk with your wife, too. She may feel responsible, believing herself undesirable, no longer attractive to you. Your wife may want to hide her body from you after surgery, because she feels disfigured and ugly. Others may be anxious and afraid of sex even after they have been assured they are in no physical danger.

Recovery is also a time when your sexual needs and hers may be in flux, along with other deeper changes: priorities, values, meaning. It is difficult to differentiate gradually changing rhythms of life from instant aging caused by pain or a cardiac event. It's possible that gradual aging is accelerated or exaggerated by a cardiac crisis - or maybe it's only your awareness that has heightened. You may have become more observant and reflective as a side effect of the crisis.

Your shifting sexual relationship is only one of the challenges you need to face together. This time of your life has the potential to be the richest and fullest yet experienced. Celebrate your time together, one day and one touch at a time. Remember, the road to success is always under construction.

Top Ten Reminders for Male Heartmates®

1. You have needs in the cardiac crisis: for information, to be needed, for support.
2. You have a right to information; it will help you make informed decisions and reduce your anxiety and feelings of helplessness.
3. Take good care of yourself - you are in crisis and recovery, too.
4. Ask for and let yourself receive support - isolation will impede your recovery.
5. Make plans for life-style changes together.
6. Fear, anxiety, depression, guilt, and anger are normal reactions to the cardiac crisis and throughout the recovery period.
7. Share your feelings with a friend or close family member.
8. Recognize and be tolerant of differences between you and your wife.
9. Talk to each other; touch each other.
10. Celebrate life *today!*

CHAPTER NOTES

1. From "Men Go to Their Caves and Women Talk," a sec-

tion of Chapter 3, pp.30 - 31, of *Men Are from Mars, Women Are from Venus*, by John Gray, Ph.D., 1992. This very readable book makes the differences, men from women, understandable. It also includes many practical suggestions about what to do once one understands. Heart disease highlights how different husbands are from their wives, and how those differences complicate recovery for the patient, heartmate, and the couple.

2. Chapter 8 in *Heartmates®* is about healing the cardiac couples' relationship. There are two major sections in the chapter: one on communication, the other on sexuality.

3. See Chapter 3, the section called "The Ogre, Anger," in this book for a more detailed description and guidance for healthy expression of anger between cardiac couples.

4. From the novel, *A Soldier of the Great War*, by Mark Helprin, 1991, p. 421.

5. If you want to read more about sexuality, see the second half of Chapter 8 in this book, "Re-pairing the Heartmate Connection." In the questionnaires sent out to male cardiac spouses prior to writing this seventh chapter, more men responded to the question about sex, indicating that their sexual lives together were "worse" since the cardiac event, than to any other question.

8

Re-pairing The Heartmate Connection

The marriage bond, symbolized by the heart in song and literature, has been threatened by the cardiac crisis. Your connection was first broken during your spouse's stay in the hospital. Once he returned home, each of you remained isolated as you tried to protect each other from undue stress.

Heart disease affects *all* relationships, including strong, loving ones. According to author and social scientist Edward J. Speedling, when a physical trauma of the magnitude of a cardiac crisis occurs, the marital relationship is challenged. "The act of healing cannot be complete until the social and emotional bonds which the illness disrupted are revitalized."[1]

The cardiac crisis draws some couples closer together, resulting in greater intimacy and support. Many heartmates' devotion to each other is enhanced. You may have become acutely aware of how much you cherish and need your mate. For other cardiac couples, the trauma pulls them apart, intensifying already existing conflicts.

You may now see even more clearly the flaws in your relationship. Unfortunately, for a few, the cardiac crisis is the final rift in an already estranged relationship.

It's not fair to blame all the imperfections in your marriage on heart disease. The patterns of your relationship were established long ago. And yet, without a doubt, the cardiac crisis has had a powerful effect. Conversely, the quality of your marriage has affected your physical and emotional recovery.

A relationship requires two partners. It's a mistake to assume that once the patient has recovered physically, the marriage is automatically healed. In order for the relationship to mend, you and your mate need to recover individually and put effort into healing the relationship. At the very least, a relationship needs to be flexible enough to adapt to a new reality that includes heart disease.

The cardiac crisis can be the catalyst for a more intimate relationship. Repairing the heartmate connection is the next logical step in your recovery after healing yourself. Honest confrontation of the changes in your relationship is a step toward deepening the marriage connection.

Communication Between Heartmates®

The value of good communication is generally recognized in our society. The cardiac crisis has undoubtedly had an impact on your communication patterns. For some couples, the disruption is minor, like assuming a quieter tone of voice. For others, more dramatic changes range from an overly polite stance to no communication at all.

Caring communication is essential for healing a wounded relationship. If you sense that the cardiac crisis has strained the communication in your relationship, speak up! As hard as it sounds, breaking the forbidding silence or shifting your conversation from safe subjects to more personal topics is the first step to improving the situation. You must first look honestly at the changes.

One way to assess change is to determine how your present communication differs from that before the cardiac crisis. Use this checklist to help you evaluate your present communication with your mate. (As you answer the questions, keep in mind how you would have responded before the crisis.)

HEARTMATES® COMMUNICATION EVALUATION CHECKLIST

Yes	No	
____	____	1. Has your tone of voice or the way you talk to your mate changed?
____	____	2. Are you careful about the words you use when you talk to your mate?
____	____	3. Are there long silences when just the two of you are together?
____	____	4. Is it difficult to keep conversation going between you?
____	____	5. Do you direct conversation away from yourselves and toward others?
____	____	6. Is your television on more than before the cardiac crisis?
____	____	7. Are you less expressive of your feelings?
____	____	8. Are you more silent about your concerns?

_____ _____ 9. Do you feel more lonely, isolated, stuck?

_____ _____ 10. Do you talk regularly about daily and long-term plans and dreams?

_____ _____ 11. Do you have permission to discuss taboo issues (life and death, sex, finances, love) since the cardiac crisis?

_____ _____ 12. Are you generally satisfied and emotionally supported by the communication you have with your mate?

A comparison of communication before and after can be useful; however, some people find it difficult to be objective and concrete about their lives. Visualization is another, more abstract way to assess changes in communication. Imagine the heartmate bond as a cord that connects you and your mate. Picture, for a moment, the symbolic flow of communication between your two hearts. How much moves through the cord? What color is the substance? Is it thick or thin, sticky or flowing smoothly? Is the passageway tight and clogged, or is the cord clean and open to the flow of communication?

This exercise can help you to see your modes of communication more clearly. If your answers reveal major changes in communication, ask yourself if these are positive or negative. The same is true for the image you summon: does it evoke a picture of the communication flow opened, severed, or somewhere in between? For some couples, the cardiac crisis provokes very serious soul-searching and sharing. Other couples become self-conscious and estranged, and, in the most extreme cases, live like strangers.

Myths to Dispel

The way you communicate is further influenced by myths. A myth is a culturally learned belief that affects your emotions and actions. As a cardiac spouse, you are particularly vulnerable to three myths.

Myth 1. It is better for the patient if you don't communicate your concerns or fears. Protection is the idea underlying this myth. When your spouse was in the hospital, rules limiting visiting hours were faithfully observed to ensure his rest. There was no way to prevent your private communication from being public. When you were allowed to visit, your time was short, and often interrupted by staff continuing their regimen of physical care.

The loss of unlimited privacy translates into the attitude that it's best just to reassure the patient with a smile, a kiss, and casual conversation. And many couples feel inhibited about expressing their affection in front of others.

As a rule, cardiac spouses believe that it's best not to worry the patient with concerns of any kind. One man proudly announced that he was taking such good care of his hospitalized wife that she had no inkling he had taken a second job to meet their medical expenses. Another cardiac spouse struggled alone with her teenage son's drinking problem, rather than solicit his father's involvement to make difficult and important decisions.

Your love for your mate, coupled with a culturally ingrained myth, is a powerful motivation to protect him. Patients' reactions to protection vary, but most feel insignificant and unessential. Finding out that Carol had made important financial decisions without asking for his input, Frank erupted angrily. "For thirty years of marriage,

I was good enough to take care of it; one little heart attack, and now I'm a nincompoop with no brain. I can't do anything around here," and he stalked out of the house.

Concealing your concerns increases the distance between you. Heart patients may not realize that their mates have difficulties of their own in a cardiac crisis. A cardiac couple sat in the hospital waiting room while their son at age thirty-eight had bypass surgery. The patient turned to his wife and asked, "Was this how it was for you when you sat waiting during my surgery? I had no idea it was so hard on this side of the knife."

Heart patients, men and women alike, lie in hospital beds worrying about the same things as their spouses. Your spouse is probably grappling with fears of dying, being disabled, and failing to provide for your family. Patients confront serious questions: Why do I have heart disease? Why did I survive? Will you still love me? Does this mean I'll die young, without seeing my children grown or my grandchildren born?

Avoiding communication about these important concerns only maintains distance. It neither alleviates the concerns nor heals the communication breakdown. Continuing to withhold feelings intensifies the isolation each of you feels. If your spouse hides having chest pain, and if you don't reveal your fears and doubts, the chasm between you will grow. Sometimes even information-bearing communication is cut off when you are estranged by the cardiac crisis. If it is too threatening to begin discussing feelings, stick to the daily concerns each of you has until you become more comfortable talking together. Decide together whether you should continue plans to redo the kitchen, where you might take your vacation, how you can help your children with their college expenses. Ask your mate where the deed to the house is located, or begin to explore the financial details of his retirement plan at work. Suggest that it would be wise to inform your children of the whereabouts of your wills and insurance policies. These topics are preliminary information for future planning for the two of you to do together.

There is no proof that avoiding communication is beneficial to a heart patient, and holding back increases your feelings of loneliness and abandonment. The relationship itself weakens without quality communication.

Myth 2. Stress is reduced by withholding anger and other negative feelings. If you believe that silence relieves stress, you may withhold your feelings. However, the exact opposite is true. Stress increases, not decreases, when we consciously withhold our emotions. Sharing them allows you to honestly let go of fear, guilt, and anger.

Communication gets stifled by withheld anger. If you bite your tongue, silently clench your fists, and replace honest feelings with bitterness or barbs, you may be camouflaging unexpressed anger. Dr. Theodore Rubin asserts that expressing anger can actually strengthen a relationship.[2] He contends that expressing anger demonstrates that a spouse cares enough to want more intimacy and is willing to invest emotional energy in the relationship. Showing your spouse your feelings requires courage because it makes you vulnerable. It is also a statement of confidence that your relationship can withstand difficulties and disagreement, and will emerge strengthened by the experience.

Ask yourself when was the last time you and your mate spoke angrily to each other. And lovingly? If it has been a while, make a commitment to start talking. Be generous in your expectations of yourself. The longer it has been since you've disclosed your feelings, the more you will need to ease back into sharing your feelings. Begin by taking small steps.

Myth 3. Good communication means agreement.
Remember, as you make tentative communication, that
everyone prefers agreement. Wouldn't it be nice if you
told your mate that you felt angry and hurt that he no
longer seemed interested in your work, and his response
was: "You're absolutely right; I'm sorry, and I'll try to show
my interest again ." While most of us would like to avoid
conflict, *people do disagree*. Disagreement is a healthy part
of a relationship. If you and your spouse agreed about
everything, your life together would be rather boring. You
could just as well have married a mirror.

Making decisions together often accentuates differences. Divergent ways of coping with a crisis can create tension and put additional stress on a relationship.
Ronald and Tina had difficulty making a decision about
his surgery. When his cardiologist recommended bypass
surgery, Ronald wanted to schedule it immediately. In her
usual inquisitive style, Tina continued to ask questions,
suggested getting a second opinion, and was generally
opposed to Ronald checking into the hospital immediately. Ron felt anxious and felt a lack of support from Tina,
while Tina said she just couldn't say "yes" when she
needed more information and time to get used to the idea.
Ron responded by refusing to consult with another doctor. Tina tried to throw the whole decision on Ron, believing that if the surgery turned out less than perfect, it
would be Ron's own fault. Without the help of a close
friend, they might not have been able to discuss their differences. Expressing their fears and their need for each
other's love enabled them to understand their differences
and reach a decision they both supported.

Learning to tolerate your mate's differences is crucial for communication. Good communication requires
more than just thoughtless talking and listening. It is the
process of making and maintaining contact with another
person.

Loving contact and clear communication are more difficult in a time of crisis. Be gentle with yourself and your heartmate as you try to improve your communication. Keep your expectations realistic, and celebrate your successes together.

Here are some "do's" and "don'ts" to help you and your mate improve communication.

HEARTMATES® COMMUNICATION GUIDELINES

DO	DON'T
Do say how you feel	Don't withdraw for fear you'll stress your mate
Do remember that your spouse has similar concerns	Don't believe the myth that communication is harmful
Do express your anger	Don't believe your re lationship is too frag ile to bear your feel ings
Do try to understand differ- ences between you and your individual style of expression mate	Don't be scared off by your mate's
Do respect your own needs	Don't forget that unspoken feelings ooze out indirectly

Do focus on loving each other	Don't avoid talking about important concerns
Do enlist help from a friend if you reach an impasse	Don't forget that communication can be difficult
Do honor individual differences	Don't mistake disagreement for disapproval

Sexuality and the Cardiac Relationship

Cardiac spouses of all ages have been affected by the sexual revolution of the 1960s. Following the publication of the Kinsey Report, people began to talk more openly about their sexuality. What before had been taboo was considered legitimate subject matter for scientific research. Despite these gains, it is still true that "nice" people don't talk about sex, at least "nice" people over the age of thirty.

For many people in your age bracket, the cardiac crisis may be the first time that you explore and discuss sexual issues. Propriety and etiquette are less important as you consider what really matters in your life. *This is a time when you both deeply need and strongly fear being connected sexually with each other.* The cardiac crisis provides the opportunity to talk about your sexuality and cultivate sexual expression with your mate.

Both men and women still have difficulty accepting their bodies. Your images about sexuality originated with parents, teachers, religious authorities, and the media. Examining your values can give you new insight into your attitudes and behavior. One cardiac spouse put it beautifully when she said, "I was never very satisfied with my body as a young woman. Now, in my fifties, I'm just beginning to discover that my body is a source of pleasure and comfort."

Not so long ago, men and women both believed that sex was something that men enjoyed and women put up with. The sexual revolution was influential in disproving that fallacy. Still, few people describe their sexual expression as a source of profound satisfaction and fulfillment.

Decades after the sexual revolution, it is still rare for medical professionals to initiate a personal discussion or actively solicit a cardiac couple's questions about the sexual aspect of their relationship. Sometimes you can find a copy of the American Heart Association's 1983 pamphlet called "Sex and Heart Disease" at your hospital or in the waiting room of your cardiac rehabilitation facility. Often, coronary care units include sex education as a part of their overall educational service for cardiac patients and spouses. But sex is still so sensitive and personal an issue that it is difficult for some professionals to be really helpful.

Only days after Marsh's heart attack, just before his release, a nurse brought a portable tape recorder and a tape to his room for us. It was a tape about sexuality and heart disease.

A strange voice came out of the machine telling me, "It was a good sign that my husband was feeling well enough to notice how attractive the nurses' legs looked." That made me angry. I wanted to scream at the voice in the immobile blue machine on the window sill, "How could you understand? I don't care if we ever have intercourse again. I'm terrified that he's going to die." Sex was the last thing on my mind right after his heart attack. And I found the tape impersonal and offensive.

We laughed sort of self-consciously together and turned it off. I felt misunderstood and wondered if my concerns about sex, or lack of concern, were unusual.

When Marsh came home and we were going to sleep together in our own bed, he put his arms around me and I fell asleep feeling secure and comforted. For some weeks sex was not a high priority.

When I did begin to think about it, my fears were overwhelming. I heard echoes from the portable tape recorder but they didn't diminish my terror. Marsh might die from the stress or excitement of an orgasm. Or maybe, at forty-three, my sex life as I had known it was over; perhaps Marsh was impotent, a side effect of his drugs. Or maybe he was disinterested because I was no longer attractive to him, or maybe it was a side effect of heart disease. Not so young and liberated that I could directly ask him about it, I kept my fear quiet, not sure how to broach the subject without humiliating Marsh and embarrassing myself.

All cardiac couples have questions about sex. There isn't anyone, regardless of any level of confidence, who doesn't have some anxiety about how heart disease will affect the sexual relationship.

There are five main misconceptions surrounding the subject of sex and heart disease. Each one contributes to feelings of fear and apprehension. They are:

1. Sexual activity is hazardous for heart patients.
2. Heart disease decreases libido and impairs sexual functioning.
3. Heart disease signifies the end of normal sexual activity.
4. Sexual prowess is the measure of masculinity, and masculinity is the measure of a male's human worth.
5. Sex is love.

None of these is true. Replace them with the truth. If you're like most cardiac spouses, you have other concerns, too. Your most pressing fear may be that your sexual relationship will be permanently damaged, destroying the closeness in your marriage. This is an absolutely natural fear, particularly in the beginning stages of recovery. In some ways it's like the first weeks after having a baby, when couples are advised to postpone sexual relations.

The early recommendation to abstain may give you the false idea that your sexual relationship is over. Although it takes some time, *the overwhelming majority of cardiac couples are physically able to resume their previous sexual relationship.*

It is generally accepted that cardiac patients experience a temporary decrease in sexual drive. There are three main reasons for the decline in libido: physical fatigue, depression, and side effects from medications. All of these factors can be treated, and usually dissipate over time.

Knowing that "this, too, will pass" doesn't necessarily diminish your fear. People in crisis also need information to help set their fears to rest. To get beyond the misconceptions, we need to examine the most current medical facts about the physical aspects of sexual activity.

Cardiac couples are fortunate because there *are* answers available, at least about male heart patients. Hopefully there will soon be a major study dealing with the sexual needs, habits, and behaviors of female cardiac patients, because women make up a growing percentage of the cardiac population.

In an article printed in the *Harvard Medical School Health Letter*, Dr. Thomas Hackett, Chief of Psychiatry at Massachusetts General Hospital and Professor of Psychiatry at Harvard Medical School, addresses many of the questions about sex raised by male heart patients and their spouses.[3]

According to Hackett, the depression that commonly follows a heart attack includes reduced feelings of sexual desire. In addition, patients in active recovery are easily fatigued and spend lots of time alone, reflecting on what has happened to them. Natural depression from trauma to the body diminishes desire. Hackett points out that for 85 percent of patients this depression (and related reduced libido) passes and never becomes a major problem. If, after three months, impotence continues, treatment is recommended.

"There appears to be no medical basis for implicating satisfying sex, in a familiar and supportive relationship, as a hazard."[4] Research done with cardiac couples who had stable, long-term relationships documented that the average amount of energy expended while having sex is equivalent to climbing two flights of stairs. To reduce your fear, watch your mate climb stairs. (I suggest you let that information sink in, and not have intercourse immediately following his climb!)

Like other physical activity, sexual participation should be resumed gradually during recovery. Dr. Hackett advises that a cardiac couple limit themselves to foreplay and abstain from intercourse for the first two to three weeks of recovery. He stresses that this is, "...not because it's dangerous but because it takes the pressure off both partners to perform. Masturbation is also perfectly safe and may ease the transition back to partnered sex. After three weeks there are usually no restrictions, though this schedule may be modified in cases of severe illness."[5] In *The Sensuous Heart*, a pamphlet from the Emory University School of Medicine in Atlanta, Suzanne Cambre, R.N., Clinical Specialist, differentiates the time restrictions for a return to sexual activity. Waiting four to six weeks is recommended for most people after a heart attack. After heart surgery the timing is the same, because it takes about that long for surgical patients to get their strength back, and for the breastbone to mend. In the absence of a heart attack, cardiac cath or balloon procedure patients have no restriction except to wait twenty-four hours for the puncture site to close.[6]

The fear of dying during intercourse should not be dismissed summarily, or without additional information. A Japanese study analyzing the cause of 5,000 sudden deaths found that of the victims, 34 died (presumably) during intercourse. Of those, 30 were with partners other than their own spouses. And virtually all had blood levels close to, or in the range of, intoxication. These data suggest that the lethal stress was not having intercourse, but that intercourse in combination with alcohol and in the context of an extramarital affair may be hazardous.

Some medications used to lower blood pressure, prevent palpitations, or control angina may, as a side effect, diminish libido or produce impotence. Drugs may affect female cardiac patients as well by reducing natural lubrication. Work with your doctor to find medications that don't have these side effects. Because of reticence on the part of professionals, it is important that the two of you be able to discuss the issue and raise it with your doctor, and that you persist until you get the answers and results you seek.

Frances, a seventy-five-year-old cardiac spouse, recalled a visit with her doctor twenty-five years ago. Usually reserved and embarrassed, Frances mustered her courage to ask him about sex. She told her physician that she and her husband had been turning their backs in bed to avoid arousing each other. Both were afraid that sexual activity would endanger his life. Their doctor emphatically informed Frances that there was no physical risk and that they could safely resume. Frances whispered shyly that it had made their last years together more precious.

Information helps us dismiss the myths. There are normal body changes that occur during sexual intercourse that have nothing to do with heart disease, nor do they put a heart patient in danger. The amount of time to have sex is between ten and sixteen minutes for average, middle-aged couples. During arousal, skin may be flushed, and breathing, pulse, and blood pressure increase. During orgasm, which lasts less than thirty seconds, the heart works the hardest. The pulse may reach 150 beats a minute, and the blood pressure may exceed 160/90. During resolution, following orgasm, the body returns to its resting rates within a matter of seconds. A heart patient may experience palpitations or angina during resolution; if discomfort lasts longer than fifteen minutes, call your doctor. For the minority of people who experience angina during intercourse, your doctor may prescribe medication for use before sex. These drugs can help prevent chest discomfort.[7]

The vast majority of patients can and do return to normal sex lives within three months of the cardiac event. The physical position adopted in intercourse appears to make no difference in the amount of stress of the sexual activity. There is no medical basis to support one sexual position being safer than another, although many cardiac couples, when the patient is the male, automatically switch to female superior position with the male underneath, thinking that a more passive posture will be less stressful.

Your comfort and confidence is far more important than your choice of positions. Falling back on what you're used to is less stressful than trying to learn new ways of being sexual right now.

If there is a problem with erection, medications should be checked. And, of course, if severe depression and/or specific sexual difficulties continue for longer than several months, consult with your doctor.

Sexuality and Self-image

It is natural for recovering male heart patients, who are coping with a changing self-image, to question their virility. The notion that masculinity is measured by sexual prowess sorely needs revision. This misconception affects male cardiac patients of all ages, adding unnecessary pressure to their physical and emotional recovery.

Hospitalized heart patients fear they are dying. Their real concerns about sexuality only begin once they feel confident about surviving. Cardiac patients who flirt with young nurses are most likely experiencing shock and denial. Nurses who respond to sexual talk at face value fail to understand the fear and insecurity resting just below the surface.

Some cardiac couples return to normal sexual activity as though nothing has happened. Sex, used as proof that "everything's fine," is only a temporary cover-up. It's confusing, when both of you know that things aren't "fine" or "just as they used to be," to pretend that everything is the same. A frank discussion of sex breaks through that agonizing pretense.

Cardiac patients may jokingly refer to themselves as "damaged goods." This usually reflects a fear of impotence, of being unable to perform like a "whole" man. If this is the case, you may hesitate to encourage your husband to return to sexual activity for fear of adding to his feelings of inadequacy. However, avoiding intimacy will only intensify the problem, and keep you both from taking that difficult but intimate step toward a healthy sexual relationship.

As a cardiac spouse, you,too, may be forced to cope with a changing self-image that affects your sexuality. A full year into recovery, one forty-nine-year-old wife of a bypass patient complained that she couldn't bring herself to be sexual very often. Although she didn't entirely understand why, she carried around an uneasy feeling that both she and her husband had suddenly gone from being young and attractive to being "over the hill." Another woman, terrified that her husband would have a heart attack in her arms, maintained a separate bedroom and refused to sleep with him at all.

Recovery may temporarily inhibit your sex life. But heart disease may not be the only factor to consider. Whether or not you have noticed, the frequency and style of your sexual relationship has changed gradually over the years. Some natural decline in frequency of intercourse is documented in people after the age of forty. The cardiac crisis may accelerate that change or bring the decline into focus.

It's unrealistic to try to maintain a standard that was established in your twenties and thirties. Television suggests that youth and speed are what counts, contributing to the pressure to perform. But maturity and comfort are equally valuable. Over time I have become accustomed to Marsh's habit of nodding off during the ten o'clock news, and, let's face it, I'm no longer able to be focused, witty, or romantic at midnight. But I relish and appreciate the softer, quieter, and more vulnerable way we embrace.

Beyond Facts About Sexuality

Following a cardiac event, some couples do have sexual problems they never had before. Most often they are related to feelings, not to physical changes or dangers. The cause does not make the problem any less real. Sexuality is a part of our deepest core. For some couples the problem stems from their interpretation of physical limitations; for others there's the fear of causing harm or the shame of being rejected. Couples may experience disinterest because of depression. Patients may be impotent as a side effect of medications, or believe that heart disease by its very nature means the end of sexuality. Solutions may be found in talking, trusting, and trying out behaviors together. Go slow! Don't be pushed from outside, the idea that it's "time to be back to normal." But don't let helplessness or hopelessness win the day either. Together the two of you can find your right balance.

Facts and information help, but they're no substitute for discussion. Be honest with your need for intimacy. It's essential. Here, as in other areas of your relationship, you will find that you and your mate differ, sometimes significantly and other times in minor ways. One of you may be eager to resume a sexual relationship, while the other may be more reticent. Be patient and kind with each other. Each of you has expectations and fears that need to be acknowledged and aired.

You are separate individuals *and* you are allies, members of the same team. Being teammates is especially essential when it comes to something so sensitive as sex. The cardiac crisis provides the opportunity to examine your changing sexual intimacy in a way that gradual aging doesn't. And for many couples, the imposed hiatus is a chance to appreciate each other and see with new eyes.

Right now, both of you need to give and receive physical comfort. Most couples are able eventually to return to pre-crisis sexual activity. In the great majority of cases, there is no medical contraindication to doing so. As time passes, changes in your mate's physical health may require further adjustments. If the severity of your mate's heart disease results in your being unable to have intercourse, it is a real loss, and one you can grieve together. If you avoid the pain or deny the need for physical intimacy and don't talk about it, your chances of turning to new, less strenuous ways of being with each other sexually are greatly diminished. In the wake of a crisis, it takes conscious effort, and some creativity, to face what is lost and find new ways to replace it.

Your sexual needs may be in flux along with other changing values and priorities. Perhaps you can be more openly appreciative of each other's affection, more direct about your needs, and more willing to give. With or without heart disease, none of us knows how long we have to live a satisfying life. If you express your love today, and you find yourself together tomorrow, you are blessed with more opportunity to live and love.

Many cardiac couples find themselves closer after the cardiac crisis than during any other period in their relationship. However, it is not unusual for cardiac spouses to confront an emotional barrier of unexpressed fear, resentment, or anger. It's hard to "make love" before those feelings are released and forgiven. Some people hold back, distrustful about depending on their mates, and fearful of disappointment. Vulnerability motivates others to work harder on their relationships. The threat of loss may ultimately open your hearts to each other. Petty irritations and aggravating differences may seem unimportant in the light of the bond heart disease has threatened.

Most couples find themselves uneasy discussing sexuality in the best of times, even when their relationship is solid and stable. A richer relationship demands the courage of both partners to talk openly about sex. Begin little by little. Tell your heartmate how wonderful it is to be held close, how much you missed the normal contact of sleeping together. Talk about your expectations and desires. There are so many ways to be intimate. Just holding hands or embracing can be enough to express caring physically. Saying "I love you" goes a long way, too.

Once you've opened up about your feelings, begin to discuss your differences respectfully and lovingly. Discuss resolutions that take both of your needs into account. Make a date to give or get a back rub, to cuddle, or to have intercourse. Scheduling time together is a way to say that your relationship has a special priority in your lives. Communication doesn't solve all problems, but conflicts and unmet needs hidden in the back of your mind can grow out of proportion. Ask each other for what you want and need. It can relieve the anguish of sexual expectations and performance anxiety.

One last misconception to debunk is the idea that sex is love. Sex is not love, although it is often mistaken for it. Cardiac couples can adapt to changes in sexual expression more easily if they have faith in the love that bonds them together. Love is experienced in many ways. Physical expressions: a touch, a kiss, a caress, sexual intercourse, are just parts of the repertoire human beings have to express themselves.

Sexual activity is more than sport, pleasure, or comfort. One cardiac spouse expressed herself this way, "Of course, sex is only the frosting on the cake - but how I love frosting." On a deeper level, it can be a way to fully experience yourself, and connect with another. Others describe sex as the momentary miracle of transcending time and space. Sex is at once the most distorted and violated, yet potentially sacred and beautiful of spiritual and physical acts. As you heal your relationship together, give sexual intercourse its correct value in your life. Do not under or overestimate its worth. Your connection to each other needs revitalization and support in order to heal. Your sexual relationship is a symbol of your love and your union. It is a way to celebrate life and your bond as heartmates.

Healing the Heartmate Relationship

Constructive and creative change requires your willingness to examine your relationship, the vulnerability to hope for increased intimacy, the compassion to forgive each other for past disappointments, and the persistence to plan and carry out the small, everyday rearrangements. You must renew your commitment to your relationship.

Sadly, there are those for whom the cardiac crisis is the event that precipitates a final breakdown of the relationship. Cindy, a thirty-seven-year-old cardiac spouse, described how she and her forty-year-old husband Jerry were, after fourteen years of marriage, considering a legal separation when Jerry suffered a heart attack. Months of recovery passed; Jerry's response to his disease was irritability and anger directed at Cindy. Her dilemma was a "Catch-22." It had been difficult enough, for all the usual reasons, to consider divorce. Could she create a new life for herself? Where would she find support when most of her family and friends were married and loyal to them as a couple? Their marriage was no longer right. But now, with Jerry's heart attack, Cindy was afraid of being cast as a selfish, irresponsible person turning her back on a sick man, like a captain abandoning a sinking ship.

No one would advise a couple to separate or divorce during recovery, because of the additional stress. Yet there are relationships that cannot be healed. Eroded trust is difficult for couples to rebuild in any situation. The cardic event, a betrayal by the body, may be experienced as a further abandonment. Usually in these cases, one or both partners have given up hope and are unwilling to put any more effort and good will into the relationship. Accept your partner's limits, and stay or go based on your own.[8] It is wise to seek professional help in such a situation to provide both of you the support and guidance you'll need to work through this major life crisis.

One of the most important elements of healing any relationship is rebuilding the trust that was shattered. The fear of being abandoned is a fundamental one all human beings live with. Cardiac spouses react in a variety of ways, from being overprotective to feigning fierce independence. Acknowledging your fear, at first to yourself and then to your mate, is a prerequisite for healing the trust between you. Your spouse can't realistically guarantee that he'll be there for you...forever. That alone is difficult and painful to admit. But once you can accept that there is no guarantee, you can begin anew, planning for a future that will include an appreciation of the ephemeral nature of life.

Whatever the state of your relationship, your challenge is to see the reality and make peace with it. Only then is there the opportunity to take advantage of new perception and understanding, and to reconnect at a level based on mutual appreciation and respect. Your marriage bond may be strengthened by sharing and surviving this experience together.

As serious and significant as your relationship is, nothing is a more powerful healer than humor. Being able to laugh at yourselves and your situation will help you see things as they truly are and enjoy your togetherness.

One of the best investments we made when Marsh was recovering from bypass surgery was a VCR. Funny movies helped us pass many hours of recuperation, but more significant, the films gave us something to laugh about, together. Marsh complained when he aggravated his incision pain by laughing too hard, but we both found it healing.

Finally, repairing the heartmate connection depends on how well the balance between the individuals' needs and the relationship's needs can be negotiated. A healthy relationship requires each partner to establish and protect individuality and simultaneously reach beyond that to care about each other. A good marriage is one in which each appoints the other guardian of his solitude.[9] *This is the most difficult challenge you face.* The cardiac crisis has made you more aware of your needs. Individual integrity means protecting your best self. Loving your mate means truly supporting and being there for him. Sometimes it's hard to see what's best. More often, it is difficult to determine how you can act in a way that honors both of you and the relationship. The wisdom of all recovery programs is to focus on one day at a time. Healing your relationship requires ongoing commitment, honesty, and love.

Once the realization is accepted
that even between the closest human beings infinite
distances continue to exist,
a wonderful living side by side can grow up,
if they succeed in loving the distance between them
which makes it possible for each to see the other whole
against the sky.[10]

Here are some suggestions that can guide you as you repair the heartmate connection.

- Share your feelings with each other.
- Let yourselves laugh and have fun.
- Cherish your time together.
- Give yourself permission to be romantic.
- Experiment with new ways to express your love.
- Make realistic plans for your future.
- Mark anniversaries of recovery.
- Celebrate being alive and together.

CHAPTER NOTES

1. Edward J. Speedling, *Heart Attack: The Family Response at Home and in the Hospital* (New York: Tavistock Publications, 1982), p. 162.
2. Theodore Isaac Rubin, M.D., *The Angry Book* (New York: Macmillan, 1969), pp. 168-169.
3. Thomas Hackett, M.D., "Men and Sex after a Heart Attack," *Harvard Medical School Health Letter*, Vol. 11, No. 5 (March, 1986), pp. 5-6.
4. Ibid., p. 6.
5. Ibid., p. 6.
6. Suzanne Cambre, R.N., B.S.H.A., *The Sensuous Heart* (Atlanta: Pritchett & Hull Associates, Inc. 1978).
7. Ibid., pp. 13, 19.
8. from *Inneractions* by Stephen C. Paul, 1992.
9. Quoted from *Letters* by Rainer Maria Rilke.
10. Ibid.

Heart Disease Is A Family Affair

A family is an extension of marriage. Connected for better and for worse, in sickness and in health. When one member of a family is wounded, each individual is indelibly scarred. Life with heart disease is truly a family affair.

A cardiac crisis deeply affects all members of your family. It is extremely traumatic for a child of any age to experience a parent's near-death. If your mate's parents are alive, they have suffered agonizing worry and pain over *their* child. Brothers, sisters, nieces, and nephews have all shared in the concern.

The cardiac crisis can also be a wonderful opportunity. Inherent within it is the potential for increased intimacy, nourishment, and support in families. Everyone is more vulnerable and sensitive. At such times, family members may drop defenses, forgive old hurts, and reach toward each other with caring and love.

Waiting during bypass surgery was excruciating.

Our thirteen-year-old daughter, Debbie, chose to be at the hospital with me rather than go to school. We sat together surrounded by several dear friends.

By midmorning I felt restless and asked Debbie to go for a walk with me. Holding hands, we made our way to an island with one tree in the urban hospital block and stood together under the sun. I suggested that we do a visualization for Marsh. We imagined the warmth and radiance of the sun entering the operating room, strengthening the surgical team, and filling the whole room with healing light. We visualized energy and prayers coming from our friends all over the country. We saw ourselves as a channel for energy flowing through us and into the hospital to Marsh and to the surgical team.

I felt especially blessed to have a child who would share such a prayer with me. Later we decided we needed another walk, so we returned to our island. With traffic whizzing by, we closed our eyes and held hands again. This time Debbie led our personal meditation.

When the chaplain brought the news that the repair had been successful and "they were closing," Debbie and I held each other, our tears of joy and thankfulness mingling. Suddenly we were starving, and we celebrated with lunch.

It is ideal when family members can support each other in a crisis. Unfortunately this doesn't always happen. A crisis can also intensify conflicts and magnify misunderstandings. The family has the basic strength and resilience of any institution that maintains itself over generations. But within all families there are painful scars and unhealed wounds. A family crisis can offer an opportunity to heal old rifts and resentments.

The cardiac crisis automatically makes you the anchor of the family. It is your task to keep relatives informed. You are solely responsible for your children: their activities, school, appointments, meals, and other arrangements. It falls on you to respond to everyone's emotional needs.

The stress of being the family anchor may not at first be obvious. But consider the weight you're carrying on your shoulders. If you're like most cardiac spouses, you're preoccupied with your mate's recovery, and you're worried about how upset your children are. You may be concerned about where the next paycheck will come from, and the last thing you want is for your children to know you're worried. You're distressed about leaving your mate's side, and simultaneously feel guilty about not giving your children enough time and attention.

Anchoring your family makes you aware that all family members are affected by the cardiac crisis. It does *not* mean that you can fix every problem or that you're responsible for healing unpleasant or painful relationships among family members. Responsible leadership means appreciating the opportunity for renewed family unity. And leadership means accepting and respecting family members' needs as they, too, progress through the cardiac crisis.

Your children's emotional needs add to your stress and exhaustion. You have to inform your child of the family crisis. Adult children should be informed as soon as possible. But even this general rule has its exceptions.

Dana feared that her daughter, Michelle, would have a miscarriage upon learning that her dad had experienced a heart attack. Michelle lived hundreds of miles away and was in the eighth month of a difficult pregnancy. Dana weighed the possible consequences of informing Michelle or withholding the information. She tried to take all factors into consideration: Michelle's need to see her father, his need to be comforted by his daughter, and the new baby's safe arrival.

Little or no attention is paid to the needs of the children of cardiac patients by school or other institutions that do provide help in cases of defined stress like divorce or the death of a parent. Unless your children openly express it, you may not be aware of what they are going through. My clients are routinely surprised when their children let them know how much the cardiac crisis has affected them.

Cardiackids are expected to be fine because their parent is recovering. In most cases, we either ignore or sweep aside children's feelings and concerns, either out of ignorance or because our own concerns are so consuming.

The cardiac crisis deeply affects children. Cardiackids have feelings they need to understand and express. They experience the fear of nearly being left without a parent, the guilt of believing they caused the cardiac event, and the shock of their secure world becoming permanently uncertain. Cardiackids need to talk out the powerful impressions and images that haunt their dreams and waking hours.

Changing Family Rules and Roles

Your position as a family anchor reaches beyond your children to members of your extended family. Relatives with whom you normally have minimal contact may be more visible than usual. Depending on how your family gets along, association with relatives can be a blessing or a burden.

As the cardiac spouse, you are the liaison for all other family members. And regardless of your relationship with individual family members, each has genuine feelings toward your mate and a real stake in his recovery. You need to protect yourself and your mate and still respect other family members' needs.

Virginia, a forty-one-year-old cardiac spouse, had difficulty keeping Lyle's family's visits to a minimum. She was worried that he wouldn't tell his three sisters and their husbands and children when he was too exhausted to visit. Even though Virginia was the youngest in the family, she was efficient and tough. She established two periods during the day when guests could come. When visiting hours were up, she personally ushered everyone out.

One morning, after being told that Lyle was napping and couldn't be disturbed, his oldest sister asked to see Virginia's cop's badge. The sister informed her, in no uncertain terms, that the family didn't appreciate being told when and for how long they could visit their own brother.

After the first three weeks Virginia loosened the rules. She was surprised when Lyle asked her to reinstate the regime, saying he was glad she had protected him. He still tired easily and found it uncomfortable to ask guests to leave.

Making decisions that take everyone's needs into account is practically impossible. You must try to be sensitive to your mate's relatives, but at times your priorities are bound to clash.

Barbara, a devoted wife, complained that her mother-in-law was sabotaging the heart-healthy diet she had instituted since Arnold's angioplasty procedure. Twice a week, *every* week, Mildred continued to deliver the home-cooked treats that she had always made to please her son. Butter-laden pastries and salty soups were Mildred's specialties. And her cooking was delicious! Barbara understood that cooking was one way for Mildred to express her love for her son. But she finally put her foot down: "Either heart-healthy recipes or no recipes."

The new dietary rules included Mildred, and there would be no exceptions.

In a family crisis, it sometimes seems as if there are too many cooks in the kitchen. Usually passive relatives suddenly become opinionated when one of their kin's health is at stake. Decision making gets complicated when affected family members differ as to appropriate action. As the cardiac spouse, the buck stops with you. You make the decisions. This demands both your assertiveness and a willingness to carefully weigh differing opinions.

Jon, a rather shy individual, described his dilemma after his wife, Lois, had a heart attack. Her family, large and vociferous, met every evening to hash over the pros and cons of Lois' treatment. When the cardiologist advised bypass surgery, Lois' family convened in earnest. Jon felt left out and impotent as they argued back and forth late into the night. They finally agreed on the "right" course of action, informing Jon that he should tell the doctor of their decision. At no point was his opinion solicited.

If you honestly believe that other family members are interfering with your mate's recovery, do whatever is needed to protect yourself and your spouse.

A word of caution: A family crisis can also be used to lay blame or to vent past bitterness. Monitoring of visiting hours or excluding close relatives from decision making - playing the cop - may disguise an unconscious desire to hurt.

Families act according to patterns that have existed and repeated themselves for generations. Each individual has unique roles in his or her family. When a family crisis hits, everyone automatically falls back on the old established roles. Sometimes these work well in helping the family cope. Or, old roles may snarl an already burdensome situation.

A thirty-two-year-old cardiackid explained how she and her sister fell into their typical roles during their mother's hospitalization. One sister was in charge of cosmetic concerns; the other handled the emotional issues. The former shopped for a new robe and nightgowns for their mother; she made sure her mom's makeup was fresh and her hair coifed to keep her spirits up. The latter translated the doctors' reports and facilitated communication among the three generations of the family.

All family members are needed during a crisis. Each member of your family is an individual with unique gifts. Appreciating each other's contributions is an essential part of pulling together. If one member of your family is best at interpreting medical information, he or she should handle that. If another has always been the clown, comic relief has its place, too. All family members, simply by virtue of their love and concern, have a valuable and legitimate role in the process of recovery.

Major Issues Confronting Cardiac Families

The effects of the cardiac crisis on family members may not be readily apparent. On the surface, your family seems the same as usual. But it's *not* the same! The cardiac crisis forces change and reversal in family relationships, roles, and rules. The long, cold fingers of uncertainty touch every family member. With the loss of certainty comes the urge to control and the yearning for order in a world suddenly strange, frightening, and uncontrollable.

If you are a parent, you are no doubt worried about the effects of the cardiac crisis on your children. The basic human fear of being abandoned, of being left helpless and alone, is an immediate as well as long-range concern for cardiackids. Since the onset of heart disease may occur in young, middle-aged, or older people, the needs of children differ from family to family. Within your family, each of your children will have individual needs depending on age, personality, and role in the family.

Your children's reactions to the cardiac crisis may evidence themselves as exaggerations of their normal behavior, or as unusual behavior that is difficult to understand. Young children may act out their fears through play. You may notice your seven-year-old play doctor or ambulance driver, her way of making order of the chaos. Children may react unconsciously with physical ailments or symptoms. A cardiac spouse described her shock when she was called by the school nurse. Her son had gone to the nurse's office with chest pains, sure that he was having a heart attack. Your ten-year-old may refuse to play with friends, suddenly becoming solicitous and parental, sensing your fatigue and vulnerability, reversing the normal role of parent and child. Your adolescent son, struggling to achieve manhood and fearful about losing his father, may take over and try to be "the man of the house." Your adult children, involved in the family business, may find decision making difficult when the authority figure is suddenly unavailable for counsel. Your independent, single daughter, usually too busy to talk, drops by every evening after work, disregarding her personal routine and social life.

Cardiac spouses will try to appear strong and competent so that their children will feel safe. You may assume a well-defended stance in order to get through the day. Ironically, when cardiackids see the facade of a strong, silent model, they get the message, "Don't ask! Don't talk about it." And they don't. This is especially true of adult children. Attuned to your stress level, they may try to cope with theirs by guarding their feelings closely. The only way children of all ages may know to be cooperative and helpful is by *not* demanding your attention, *not* rocking the boat.

Unexpressed feelings can fester and leave permanent scars. Once a cardiackid is shaken by the knowledge that his parent is mortal, he will never again be an innocent. The illusion of security is forever broken.

Edward, age fifty-eight, was twelve years old when his father suffered a heart attack. Whenever Edward and his brother made the least bit of noise, their mother would come out of the kitchen or bedroom, looking frightened, and say, "Shhh, shhh." Edward was terrified that his noise would kill his father. He became more and more withdrawn.

Recalling those days, Edward remembered that his family never talked about his father's illness or what was happening to them. One evening at the supper table his fear erupted. His question echoed through the kitchen. "Will Daddy die?" His mother pushed her chair away from the table and ran crying into the bathroom. The rest of the family finished supper in silence.

After more than forty years, Edward's memories are still vivid. The trauma of having been a cardiackid returned when his wife Florence had a heart attack. Once he shared his memories and feelings, he was able to cope with the present. Florence's heart attack was an opportunity for Edward to heal an old wound.

Role Reversals

Changes in family relationships occur as a result of the cardiac crisis. If the onset of heart disease means that the cardiac patient does not return to work, financial issues may affect the family dynamics. When adult children begin to help parents financially, it is the beginning of the role reversals that come with aging. Parents, used to being in charge, have to adjust to being progressively more dependent on their children.

Margaret, a cardiac spouse, was concerned about her eleven-year-old son. Ever since Rob's dad suffered a heart attack, Rob had assumed responsibility for all the physical work around the house. Snow-shoveling is a major undertaking in their northern winter.

On the surface such a change in family responsibility seems simple and uncomplicated. Each winter tensions arise in the family. Rob's dad feels guilty that he is physically unable to shovel and must leave the entire job to Rob. He paces from window to window, scrutinizing Rob, watching every flake he moves. When he's finished, Rob saunters in, proud of the job he's done, hoping he will hear praise from his dad. His father, unable to express his guilt, either criticizes the quality of Rob's work, or comments on how he ought to have done it. The scene usually ends with Rob slamming the door to his room and isolating himself for the rest of the day. And since each year brings new snow, winter continues to be a stormy time, symbolizing the changes that heart disease has brought their family.

Less dramatic but just as painful is the change of life-style as aging parents become more dependent on grown children who are busy with their own families and careers. Sunday dinners and holiday celebrations, long the pride of the parents, move down to the next generation. Children may need to arrange for their parents' doctor visits, transport them when they can no longer drive, and take charge of their Sunday outings.

The stress of this transition is difficult for all family members. Children may take over tasks lovingly or grudgingly, and parents may give them up graciously or stubbornly. All of these changes can be difficult to face and accept. Professional counseling can help improve coping and communication skills.

Many cardiac couples find it a difficult adjustment to accept help, especially from their children. For most of us, giving is easier than receiving. You and your mate may find yourselves in the "sandwich generation," between your grown children and your aging parents. When your focus and energy are directed toward coping with the cardiac crisis, carrying the responsibility for aging parents adds more stress to an already overwhelming situation.

If you are sandwiched between aging parents and growing children, you need to decide where to put your energy. You may be accustomed to the role of caregiver, but with the additional energy required to deal with the cardiac crisis, you may be unable to give as much as usual to your children or your parents. The young and the aged may be unprepared or unable to give you the care you need right now.

Don't be reluctant to ask for help from other members of the extended family at this time. *You cannot do it all yourself!* And members of your immediate family need to give, too. Even young children can make worthy contributions and find comfort in being needed. Other sources of help are available through your local social service agencies. Don't hesitate to ask for the assistance of the social worker at your hospital to connect you with the appropriate agency.

Dealing with Cardiackids

Your love for your children makes you naturally

concerned about their reaction to the cardiac crisis. Perhaps you feel that you must be more in charge than usual in order to compensate for their feelings of insecurity. You are the one who will assume the role of intermediary between your children and your sick spouse, keeping each filled in on how the other is doing during hospitalization. Reassured by the safe return of a parent from the hospital, children may begin to express negative feelings of fear or anger over what they experienced as abandonment and neglect. Less able to speak directly about what's bothering them, children's reactions may take the form of poor school performance, inability to get along with siblings, or becoming depressed or accident-prone.

Juggling your needs for privacy and support with your children's increased demands is a tricky balancing act. You want to be there for them at a time when you are struggling to be there for yourself.

The impulse to protect your children from pain and anguish is universal. But the truth is, it's impossible to do so. The cardiac crisis has occurred. You, your mate, *and* your children have been and will continue to be affected. Even if you could protect your children from hurt, it wouldn't necessarily be doing them a favor. Learning how to cope in a crisis is a valuable part of growing up.

There is no such thing as a perfect parent. And the pressure of being a cardiac spouse makes parenting even more challenging. If you're not as patient and responsive as usual, keep in mind that you have been parenting alone, without your main source of support, your mate.

My rule of thumb in dealing with children is to remember that *kids are people*, too. In a cardiac crisis, children have questions and they have feelings. A child of any age has the right to be informed about what is happening to his or her parent.

Your Children's Right to Know

Adult children don't have the same access to hospital staff that you do. They aren't around as much as you are, and doctors and nurses may not take their questions seriously. Hospital regulations might prohibit young children from visiting at all.

Nothing is more fearful than the unknown. Even though you may not understand the details of every conversation you have with the medical staff, you do experience some relief from being given regular progress reports and information. Your children may not understand every detail either, but they will feel included and reassured if they are also informed.

Sometimes children get the idea that they are superfluous or in the way during the cardiac crisis. If you keep them apprised of discharge plans and recovery programs, they will feel more free to ask other questions they might have.

You are the natural liaison between your children and your spouse. At times this arrangement may offer the only option. But nothing is as satisfying as direct contact between them. As soon as your mate is moved from cardiac care to a recovery unit in the hospital, you can arrange daily phone communications between him and his young children. Calls need not be long, but it is affirming and encouraging to hear daddy's voice. Sharing a goodnight kiss over the phone is better for both than none at all.

Over the long term, it is important for you to step away from negotiating family relationships. Trying to improve others' relationships doesn't work. You may be tempted to step in and help when you see your spouse and your adult children striving to establish communication. They may have conflicts to resolve, new things to talk about, or love to express to each other. If there is stress or enmity between your mate and your children the cardiac crisis may ignite it. You face the impossible paradox: maintaining your alliance with your mate while simultaneously protecting your children, the most basic and instinctive parental act. Give them the space to work out their relationships without your interference.

Questions from your children for which you have only tentative answers or none at all can distress you. Inviting your children's questions does not mean that you know the answers. Feel free to respond with three simple words, "I don't know."

The most feared question, of course, is, "Is my daddy going to die?" The truth is that you don't know for sure. You might want to cloak the issue and respond only with the data and statistics that you have heard at the hospital. But a real question needs an answer from your heart as well as your mind. Your response might be, "Chances are, since Daddy has lived through the first forty-eight hours after a heart attack, that he will recover. I sure hope so, although I don't know for sure, and even the doctors can't be certain. I know that you're really scared and I feel afraid, too." Such an answer may be followed by a long hug, shared tears, a special prayer.

What if you are ready and willing to answer your children's questions, but they remain silent? The most effective way to respond is to be open and accessible. Forcing children to talk about their feelings will only make them more resistant. Each of your children will deal with the cardiac crisis in an individual way.

Our family had a week to plan before Marsh's bypass surgery. Debbie decided immediately that she wanted to be with me in the hospital. She said she would be unable to concentrate and would find it intolerable to be sit-

ting in school while her dad was being operated on.

Our fifteen-year-old son, Sid, reacted in an opposite way. He thought it would be unbearable to sit in the hospital for hours. His preference was to be at school and be distracted from the surgery.

Sid worked out an elaborate plan for being informed. His idea was to run home from school and hear the phone ringing as he unlocked the front door. We agreed on the exact minute that I would call, and we synchronized our watches. And that was how Sid received the news that his dad had come through the surgery successfully.

I was surprised at how differently our two children reacted. I particularly appreciated that each of them knew exactly what they needed on that stressful day.

Your children may tell friends their account of what happened to them and their parent during the cardiac event. You know from your own experience that telling and retelling your story is a necessary review that helps you integrate and understand what happened. Your children's versions of the experience may be very different than yours. Restrain, if you are able, the urge to "correct" them.

As they share their feelings, you may feel it's up to you to "make your kids feel better." You don't have the power to do that. You can only trust the storytelling process to help your children come to a sense of order and peace about such confusing and chaotic experiences.

Helping Your Children Heal

Children need to be encouraged to speak about the frightening images they have. Like telling a nightmare, bringing the dark and frightening memory into the light is important. Such images may never be forgotten, but saying them aloud can help divest them of their power.

When given the opportunity, most cardiackids are eager to talk about their experiences and images. One young man said that he couldn't get free from the horrible image of his mom straining against the respirator. A teenager described her pain and shock seeing her father so vulnerable in the cardiac care unit after a heart attack. An adult cardiackid explained his paralysis in decision making in the family business because his image of his father was of the perfect businessman. He was sure that he would make an irreversible mistake. He confronted his feelings of inadequacy as he moved toward the inevitable, the younger generation taking over the work of the patriarch.[1]

Rarely do cardiac families talk about how the cardiac patient looked after open heart surgery. The sounds of the respirator and the numerous monitoring devices; the sight of countless tubes coming in and going out of the patient's body, neck, and nose; the antiseptic smells and the chill of the patient's flesh are too much to assimilate. The technology may be sophisticated, and the techniques may be routine, but when a spouse and children of any age see their loved one in this state they may respond with horror, terror, or despair. If the unspoken rule is to "say nothing" or "keep a stiff upper lip," each family member suffers alone.

A cardiac spouse expressed concern that for months her nine-year-old son, Bobby, cried every time he heard an ambulance siren. I suggested she ask him what the sound reminded him of, and that she respond to Bobby from her heart. Bobby told her that the sound reminded him of seeing his daddy being taken away in the dark night by a screaming ambulance. He didn't think he would ever see his dad again. Bobby sat on his mom's lap and they had a long hug. Then they talked about how scary that time had been for everyone in the family, and how lucky they all were that Dad had recovered. Happily, after their talk, Bobby stopped crying at the sound of a siren.

Making yourself available to share your feelings with your children can be a relief for all of you. There is no need to hide your honest emotions. Expressing your feelings openly is an act of courage; encourage your children to do the same. Shared family tears soothe and heal.

Children in cardiac families may need an expanded foundation of support during the cardiac crisis. If you have children of school age, I recommend you tell your children's teachers about the cardiac crisis. Information that deepens a teacher's understanding of what occupies your child's thoughts is useful. Your child's teacher can be a symbol of stability during a time of emotional confusion and family change. An adult ally outside the family can be a teenager's supportive listener.

Informing teachers may include educating them about the cardiac crisis, telling them that it *is* a family crisis, even though cardiac recovery is expected. Remember, bypass surgery has come to be seen as routine - with over 500 bypass operations done every day in the United States, it is our most common surgery. And as the frequency of angioplasty procedures surpasses surgery, we grow even more accustomed to thinking of these treatments as ordinary. Recovery from heart attacks is thought to be occasion for celebration and gratitude. Let the teachers know that your children are experiencing a family crisis. Each family member is in the process of understanding and accepting a new reality; such change requires time and patience. Children have serious questions and experience feelings that need to be encouraged and supported by sensitive adults.

Carla visited her daughters' parochial school when Patrick needed bypass surgery. She wanted the teachers to be prepared for their girls' reactions. Carla was pleasantly surprised to find that her eight-year-old, Marie, had already told her teacher. In fact, she had asked that a special prayer for her dad be included in the regular morning prayer. Next, Carla visited her ten-year-old's teacher. The teacher knew nothing about the family crisis and was glad to be informed so she could be helpful. Carla returned home confident that the girls' teachers, now informed, would do what they could to listen and provide reassurance without minimizing the girls' concerns.

Dealing with young, and grown, children over time requires a basic understanding of the nature of the cardiac crisis. Although your children are different from you, each a unique individual, they will go through a similar process as they cope with the cardiac crisis. Universally, family members experience disruption, shock, confusion, anxiety, fear, depression, and anger, and eventually accept a new family life that includes heart disease. They may exhibit and express their reactions differently, but they, too, are recovering from a crisis.

It takes time for cardiackids to come to terms with heart disease in the family, but children naturally and gradually return to normal behavior. In some cases, however, the cardiac event results in more serious long-term problems.

What are danger signals that indicate your child is stuck in the crisis and needs help? Because each child is unique, it is not easy to define normal progress. Take into account how long particular behavior continues, and how your child's actions differ from before the cardiac crisis. Remember that you know your child better than anyone. If you sense that he or she is having serious problems, trust your judgment. Here are some warning signals:

Angry, rebellious outbursts

Dramatic changes in their marks at school
Behavior problems at school
Persistent nightmares
Eating or sleeping problems
Lethargy and/or exhaustion
Belligerent and/or argumentative behavior
Alcohol or drug problems
Clinging to parents
Crippling fears
Withdrawal and/or isolation

If you believe your child is suffering from any one or a combination of these behavioral signals, don't hesitate to consult a school social worker or psychologist. Another resource is your local hospital's social service department. You may find that there are professionals or programs available to your child at school or at the hospital. Many high schools have groups for students who are experiencing unexpressed grief or family stress. Expert advice doesn't supplant your influence; it supplements it.

Here is a guide to help you evaluate your family members' needs as they deal with the cardiac crisis. It includes reminders and hints to improve communication within the family. You will also find suggestions for getting help and support for your family.

HEARTMATES® FAMILY NEEDS ASSESSMENT GUIDE

1. Does each family member know that it is normal for *all* family members to be affected by the heart disease of *one* of its members? If not, how can such an understanding come about?

- Get more information.
- Ask more questions.
- Have more discussion among family members.
- Express feelings.
- Share this guide, chapter, or book with family members.

2. How aware and supportive are you to each of your children's reactions to the cardiac crisis? You might want to think about the initial and long-range reactions of each family member. Remember, no response is better than any other. Here is the perfect moment to value and appreciate the individual qualities of each member of your family.

3. Do family members ask questions and comment on concerns that are important to them individually within the family? If not, how can this need be met? Here are some suggestions to help relax the code of silence that may exist within your family:

- At your next family get-together (Sunday dinner, a visit, or a prearranged family meeting) ask directly if anyone has questions about your spouse's present condition, past cardiac events, or future plans.
- Establish a question box in the kitchen that can be opened regularly at a time when all family members are present. Let questions be asked anonymously, if family members aren't able to ask aloud.
- Be willing to share your questions, too. You don't have to understand it all perfectly. Other family members may be able to offer new perspectives.

4. How do you inform your children about the difficulties you are having?

- Do you say how you feel?
- Do you ask them to listen to you?
- Do you solicit their opinions and advice as you confront necessary and difficult decisions?
- Do you allow your children to give to you (physically, emotionally, financially)?

5. Does each family member have someone outside the family to talk to regarding the cardiac crisis? Is the listener available often, regularly, or seldom? Is the listener an extended family member, a friend of approximately the same age, a special adult, a mentor, a spiritual guide?

6. Have you let others offer support to you and your family?

- Inform your children's teachers.
- Let your minister, rabbi, or priest know of your family crisis.
- Contact your hospital cardiac rehabilitation staff to get support for family issues.
- Seek help from a family therapist or social service agency specializing in family concerns.

Simply wanting your family to become more intimate isn't enough to make it happen. Family patterns are established over long periods of time, often passed down through generations. Consequently, change is slow - one step at a time. Even positive change includes the element of uncertainty, so it can be strange and, in some ways, rather frightening.

During the process of recovery, anything uncertain can feel threatening. Go slowly. And remember: You alone are not responsible for all the other members of your family. As much as you may want the cardiac crisis to be a catalyst for closeness, you can't make other people change. They have to be motivated, too. Concentrate on how you can be available to give and receive from members of your family.

Concerning Blended, Broken, and Alternative Families

Heart disease does not confine itself to the ideal American family, a loving couple with 2.4 children. It strikes blended families, separated and divorced couples, and couples who are not married. These family configurations complicate an already complex situation. Family therapists say that once there are children, there is no such thing as divorce. Events that have an impact on families - and surely heart disease is one of these - mark all family members, past and present.

SEPARATION AND DIVORCE

As a former spouse of a cardiac patient, your concerns will run the gamut from responding emotionally to your ex-spouse's heart disease to wondering how to help your children. You probably have at least some of the following questions: Shall I visit at the hospital? Why do I feel sad, angry, or afraid when we're no longer married? Is it appropriate for me to share my feelings with the patient? With our children? How should I act in relation to his family? How can I interact with his present spouse? What is the most supportive position I can take for our children in a family crisis from which I'm isolated, or about which I have unresolved feelings?

My advice in these matters is simple, but not necessarily easy: Act from your heart! There are no right or wrong answers. Etiquette and protocol don't reach into this realm. If there is anything unresolved between you and your ex-spouse, there may be criticism no matter what you do.

Try not to judge or censor your feelings. Ambivalence is normal in this situation. You are entitled to respond any way that seems right. You may also decide to use the opportunity of the cardiac crisis to reconcile old differences. That is perfectly appropriate. Hard feelings may soften at a time when heart disease has made all of you more vulnerable. And then again, nothing may change between the two of you.

No matter how you feel toward your ex-spouse, try your best to respect your children's relationships with him or her. If your children's loyalty has been a point of contention, a family crisis can escalate it. Your children's love should not be something to fight over. Children should never have to shoulder the burden of your pain and anger with each other. They have a right to their own personal relationship with each of you.

If you feel unwelcome or too awkward to visit at the hospital or at home during recovery, call a member of your ex-spouse's family to arrange a visit for your children. It may be hard to accept that your children need something that you aren't in a position to give, but there's more to being a good parent than meeting their every need. If that is the case, arrange for them to connect with grandparents or aunts and uncles who can function as their confidantes or provide them the "warm fuzzies" such a difficult situation requires.

UNMARRIED HEARTMATES®

If you are a heartmate outside the legal bond of marriage, your situation poses questions of a different sort. Family members who rally round your sick heartmate may not even know about you or that your relationship exists. If they do, they may not appreciate the nature of your relationship or realize that you are deeply affected by your heartmate's illness.

If your relationship is a secret, your contact may need to be clandestine or even temporarily cut off. The cardiac crisis may be an opportunity for the two of you to consider the emotional costs of keeping your relationship from your families. Since heart disease is incurable, and potentially life-threatening even when recovery is complete, you may consider a change in the terms of your relationship.

Also to be discussed are financial arrangements for your future. Financial planning may change due to the cardiac crisis. If your heartmate has been providing financial support, it may be impossible for this to continue. Going through a cardiac crisis may give rise to new values, affecting the way you deal with money in your relationship.

Your participation in giving your heartmate physical and emotional support during recovery is more difficult if you are unmarried. If your loved one is part of his own family, your visible involvement in his recovery probably won't be welcome. If you are openly involved with, but not living with, a cardiac patient, the logistics of maintaining two households make support more complicated.

As an extralegal cardiac spouse, you will be doing your grieving and adapting without the safety or foundation that a family normally provides. No matter the reason why you've not married, you suffer during the cardiac crisis like all heartmates do. Seek out people who can be supportive to you, and who will listen to your concerns. Professional counseling is a practical aid when your needs require confidentiality.

Family Heartache

When a family gets stuck in the process of recovery - when communication is essentially shut off, so that issues are not being confronted - natural healing doesn't happen.

The scenario of a "stuck" family may resemble the following story: Several months of recovery have passed. Father, the cardiac patient, feels depressed and is irritable and demanding. Mother, the cardiac spouse, feels resentment and is fatigued and overworked. The eldest daughter, who temporarily dropped out of college when her father suffered his heart attack, has neither looked for a job nor made arrangements to continue her schooling. The second child, a sixteen-year-old high school junior, is coming home late at night. His sullen and silent style has become exaggerated, and his grades have fallen. The youngest child, an eleven-year-old girl, is afraid to go to bed without a light on, and is often heard crying or screaming with nightmares.

No one mentions what is happening to any one individual in the family. No one notices that the family as a unit is failing to support its members. The crisis seems to have fragmented the family system and the children are acting out the pain that Father and Mother have neglected to address.

Sometimes school will call attention to a symptom by reporting falling grades or by commenting on behavioral changes in a child. It is a mistake, however, to focus on a child, officially labeling a symptom of family dys-function as an individual problem or illness. Instead, the cardiac couple should be encouraged to face the issues directly. If they can, the children will be liberated from the obligation of carrying the unexpressed anger and pain of their parents.

Short-term consultation with a family therapist is the most appropriate help for a cardiac family. The fam-ily therapy perspective will protect an individual family member from becoming the erroneous focus, obscuring the real family issues opened by the cardiac crisis. Brief intervention is frequently all a family needs to break through the code of silence.

When parents are able to relate how frightened they are about having heart disease or how grateful they are for recovery, it has magical effects on all family mem-bers. When everyone acknowledges fear, the chance that their hearts will open to each other increases exponen-tially, and the family can become a secure place for ev-eryone. In a safe environment, family members can ask their questions and can voice their feelings.

The cardiac crisis offers more than just an oppor-tunity to test a family's power to withstand and ward off pain. When hearts are physically and emotionally wounded, as all hearts are in a cardiac family crisis, there is a chance for the basic strength of the family to grow and for love to expand.

Not all families need professional help. A technique that can help is visualization. Here is a Heartmates® ex-ercise that you can do alone, or you can invite your fam-ily to participate. Have someone read the exercise aloud each time you do it to avoid interruption, or tape the in-structions yourself. Make sure to pause to give yourself time to experience each part of the visualization.

HEARTMATES® VISUALIZATION:
A HEALING FAMILY MEETING

Find a quiet and comfortable place to sit. Close your eyes. Let yourself breathe normally. Relax. Imagine that with each inhalation you breathe in energy and with each exhalation you let go of tension. Continue to focus on your breathing until you feel calm and alert.

Now imagine a room in your home that is the warmest and most comfortable for your family. It may be your kitchen, den, or porch. Notice its furnishings and what makes it warm. See it awaiting and welcoming your family. And now, in your mind's eye, see all your family seated in a circle in this comfortable room. Everyone seems to know why they're here. The atmosphere is hopeful and cooperative.

You begin your family meeting by everyone holding hands as you sit in a circle. Together you share a silent prayer of gratitude for recovery, and a petition for family cohesion and individual strength. As much as you can, experience the feeling of all of you together in this moment of silence. As you complete the prayer, everyone drops hands, and an atmosphere of respect and concern settles over the room. There is a sort of peace, an aura of acceptance and protection that falls over the family.

Now imagine that without blame or shame, each family member speaks in turn about one personal concern. You listen with your heart to what each family member says. You, in turn, hear your own contribution with your heart as well. There is no verbal response to any statement that is made, but there is respect in the listening and there is caring from each to all.

Imagine that as each person speaks, the weight of the family is lightened and the light in the room gets brighter. The air the family is breathing is fresh and clean. You can smell growing grass and blossoming flowers.

Now, as the meeting ends, you sense family members really seeing one another. Each member is respectful of other family members' rights and abilities to deal with the crisis in their own ways and by their own timetables. Some affection may be expressed.

Everyone agrees to meet again soon. Your favorite room empties; you experience realistic hope about your family's ability to cope with the cardiac crisis.

You again focus your attention on your own breath. Gradually return to your present reality. Continue to breathe fully and naturally. Return, renewed, to the present.

Recovery and Hope for the Cardiac Family

How can you see opportunity in the cardiac crisis? "In the light of our everyday world, we cannot see the stars."[2] So much of your energy goes into just coping with the minute-to-minute and day-to-day changes. Everything you wish is focused on the past: You wish this had never happened, that the family would return to normal. Recovery and healing is a natural part of the cardiac crisis, too.

The power of the cardiac crisis has jolted and shocked everyone. Each member of the family needs to recover, and the family as a whole needs to heal. What can you do? The essential elements of every recovery include communicating, expressing feelings, understanding the meaning of the crisis, and supporting one another through the grieving process. Build an environment that honors individual differences and permits each person his own responses. Make space for every family member to cooperate.

For all families and each family member, the cardiac crisis means something different, and the pace of a family's healing is also unique. Your family will move at its own rate and in its own way toward recovery.

The cardiac crisis can be regarded as an opportunity for reconnection within the family. A crisis can strengthen family bonds. Being there for one another puts "heart" into the family. Participation will enhance respect and deepen trust among cardiac family members.

A Note to Cardiackids

As a cardiackid, your special concerns are different from your parents'. Perhaps you have been fortunate in having someone outside the family to talk with about the changes that are taking place. Or maybe you feel confused and alone. As a counselor and the mother of two teenage cardiackids, I offer you the following guidance:

1. You have a right to know what is happening. Depending on your age and your role in the family, you may or may not have been given sufficient information about what is going on. You are entitled, no matter how old or young you are, to know your parent's condition and prognosis. The cardiac crisis is real; your life is affected. *Ask the questions you need answers to.* You may have to ask your parents because you don't have direct access to doctors and other professional personnel. If you can't get the answers from your parents, ask others in your family - older brothers and sisters, cousins, aunts and uncles. There is nothing more difficult than dealing with the unknown. Some things just can't be known or predicted, but you should get whatever information exists. It is okay to ask any question that you have, even if there isn't an answer available. Remember to ask your questions again later, or to go to someone else if you don't get a satisfactory answer the first time.

2. Accept your feelings and find ways to release them. All the feelings that you experience are normal. Most cardiackids have different feelings at different points of the crisis. You may go back and forth between feeling sad and happy, afraid and anxious, embarrassed and ashamed, helpless and jealous, depressed and ambivalent, angry and guilty. All of these feelings are okay.

If your family is one that is uncomfortable talking about feelings, find other constructive ways to express yourself. Keep a diary or a journal and regularly write about how you feel. Talk with your friends. Search for an adult who will listen to you. Perhaps your favorite teacher, coach, or an activity leader whom you respect will take the time to hear you out. At a time like this, your special relationship with a grandparent or favorite relative can be good for both of you.

It really is important for you to express your feelings. Keeping them locked up inside can freeze the natural development of your relationships with your family and other people, too.

3. Don't blame yourself. Cardiackids sometimes believe that their behavior caused their parent's illness. That is not true! If you blame yourself, you will act overly careful and withhold your feelings - and that won't help anyone. If somebody tells you that you can cause a fatal heart attack by making a lot of noise, or that angering the patient will do him harm, don't believe it. Your feelings and behavior cannot cause a heart attack.

4. Don't be ashamed. If you believe that your parent is damaged or different because of heart disease, you may feel embarrassed by or ashamed of that parent, your family, even of yourself. You also love your parent, and feel guilty about having such negative thoughts. Ambivalent feelings are both normal and confusing as you heal from the cardiac crisis. But having a disease, or having physical limitations, doesn't make a person less whole. All human beings have dignity and deserve respect, regardless of their physical form. (This truth is illustrated in the films *The Elephant Man* and *Mask*.)

5. It takes a while to return to normal thinking and functioning after a crisis. The cardiac crisis will affect you in ways you might not expect. You may have problems paying attention in class long after your parent is home from the hospital. Plan for more time than usual to do your homework. If you find that you can't think clearly, don't push yourself. Stop studying and go for a bike ride, shoot some hoops, talk on the phone, or take a warm shower. When you go back to the books, be gentle with yourself. You may even want to get permission from your teachers to turn some assignments in late. I'm not suggesting that you use the cardiac crisis to procrastinate or to get special privileges. Taking good care of yourself may require you to ease some of the stresses that you would handle effectively under normal conditions.

6. Roles and responsibilities in the family are changed by the cardiac crisis. You may be aware of the typical role that you and your brothers and sisters play in your family. If you are the "good child" in the family, you may find yourself really "wiped out" from taking on extra tasks and jobs to help your parents. If you are the "shy one" in the family, you may find it hard to get the information you need and even harder to talk about how you feel. Most people fall back on their typical roles to get through a crisis. It is not the best time to experiment with a new way of interacting with your family, but go for it if you can. A crisis is a time when everything is anything but familiar, so it is possible to try new modes of relating.

You also are likely to notice that your parents' roles have switched, maybe temporarily and maybe permanently. Your dad may have taken over the kitchen since your mother's surgery. Or Mom may have become more of a disciplinarian since Dad was hospitalized. Your parents may be struggling with new and different responsibilities and may seek your help. You may have to get up early before school to shovel the driveway, or take over the jobs your dad usually does, like changing screens and storms on the windows of your house.

New responsibilities, even temporary ones, can make you feel terrific. It is natural to care when your family is in crisis, and you can show some of that by being responsible and helpful. Putting a younger brother to bed, cleaning up the kitchen, or mowing the lawn is just exactly what you need to do to show your parents you care. Such tasks are practical and measurable and can give you the reassuring sense that the family can count on you when so much seems strange and confusing. Household tasks also give you a way to help your changing family. On the other hand, you may resent having to take on extra responsibility, especially if you don't have any say in the matter, and no one acknowledges your efforts.

In an ideal family all of these changes would be discussed and accepted before they happened. But no family is ideal, and it is more likely that you are assigned, sometimes without words, responsibilities that may burden you.

7. Try to understand your parents. Conflict between your parents may have escalated since the cardiac crisis. Their differences and different reactions to the crisis increase the tension between them. Whether they tell you so or not, it is important for you to know that they also feel helpless, out of control, frightened, sad, and angry about the cardiac crisis.

8. It is not your responsibility to take care of your parents. Even though you may want to alleviate the tension that you feel within the family, *you can only change yourself. You can't change other people.*

If your parents are separated or divorced, you may feel caught in a loyalty bind. You may live with your mother and depend on her to take you to see your father. It is an awkward situation, but one in which you owe it to yourself to do what your heart tells you. Staying close to your cardiac parent is your right, even if you no longer live together. Discuss the situation with both your parents, letting them know that you love them both.

The deeper questions you must wrestle with concern your loss of innocence. You have seen that your parent is mortal, and now, the one thing you thought was secure, isn't. If your parent can die, then nothing in life is for sure. Remember when you realized there was no Santa Claus or Tooth Fairy? Your disappointment and sadness were real then - and they are now, too. You need time and space to mourn the loss of what you believed. Once you do that, you will have the opportunity to develop a more realistic foundation on which to build new trust. And that may lead you to appreciate just how precious your family and life itself are.

Our son, Sid, was a senior in high school when he wrote the following essay. His assignment was to write about an event that had influenced his life. Sid rarely communicated his feelings verbally with the family. I had no idea that his father's heart disease had caused so profound a change in him. His essay was proof to me that images and memories need to be expressed if we are to overcome their hold on us. Cardiackids need to express their feelings in their own way, and in their own time. I was awed and moved as I witnessed Marsh's and Sid's hugs and tears after Sid read his essay to us one evening in our kitchen.

HE AIN'T HERCULES, HE'S MY FATHER

A soft placid sheet of snowflakes filled the skies on the cold winter evening. The scream of the ambulance snapped the peaceful hush of the night, but quickly became muffled. The screams remained in my mind long after. The ambulance held my father in its hollows while he fought for his life with a heart attack. Only minutes before, we were all sitting together watching "Monday Night Football." Now my mother, sister, and I were watching the ambulance disappear into the night. Although I had always loved him, I never realized how valuable my father was to me until I almost lost him.

At age fourteen, I "loved" my father because he was my dad; it was no more than the normal feeling a son has for his father. Nevertheless, he was my hero, and I looked up to him as a boy does to his favorite sports star. In high school, my father captained three sports: football, basketball, and baseball. He was the "All-city" quarterback and was voted the best athlete by his class. Through his mid-forties, he remained physically active, participating in softball, racquetball, and golf. He not only instructed me in the fine points of baseball, he also taught me how to wrestle by pinning me weekly during our "roughhousing matches." From my perspective, he was as close to Hercules as a man could get. I never had a foreshadowing of the disastrous event.

The hospital room was only steps away. I slowed my pace, afraid to see my wounded father. I peeked in and saw him: lifeless, with tubes going in and out of his body. His eyes opened when I entered the room, and when he made an effort to smile, I broke into tears. I could not believe that my hero was crippled. He was too weak to lift his hand to hold mine, so I grasped his hand and I held him, all of him, for the first time in my life. At that point, I realized how much I loved him! He was a supernova, an exploded star that had become thousands of times stronger and brighter.

After his hospitalization, my father returned home and didn't leave the house for another month. With my hero gone, a new relationship with my father dawned. His body had failed him; as time passed, he started to adjust. I learned what true disappointment was by watching the pain that he went through; it hurt inside to see him short of breath after climbing a flight of stairs.

Because of the threat that any day he could be gone forever, I have learned to value his presence whenever I am with him. I no longer take his "being there" for granted. No more do I worship my father as a hero. Rather, I observe with new eyes and have a greater understanding of who he really is. I watch him make mistakes, and I note his shortcomings. We discuss our daily lives, share humor, and compare our beliefs. My hero is gone. But I have a deeper feeling of love for the man that took his place.

CHAPTER NOTES

1. See the chapter, "How Devastating Illness Devastates The Family," in Maggie Strong's *Mainstay: For The Well Spouse of the Chronically Ill* (Boston: Little, Brown & Co., 1988).

2. Jean Shinoda Bolen, M.D., *The Tao of Psychology, Synchronicity, and the Self* (SanFrancisco: Harper & Row, 1979), p. 2.

10

Opening Your Heart

The cardiac spouse experience may seem largely a matter of coping. Six months . . . a year . . . five years down the road, you may remember this as the time you had to take care of business and try to get along the best you knew how. The countless adjustments, from medical decisions to changes in life-style, consumed your energy, attention, and time.

The cardiac crisis turned you in on yourself. Becoming more introspective and self-centered is a normal and instinctive means of self-protection. Your world got very tiny, as you concentrated on coping with your personal issues.

*In 1977 a friend recommended that I read the book, **Alive**, a true story about the survivors of a plane crash in South America. I didn't recall ever hearing or reading about the crash in the news. When I opened the book, I was surprised to find that the date of the crash was the same day as my mother's funeral. At first I felt embarrassed* *about being so out of step, and wondered what else I had missed, being so absorbed in my personal pain. But when I thought about it, I could understand the natural tendency for energy to flow where it is most needed. I imagine it's the same when white cells rush to a wound at a specific location in the body to provide the additional help needed for healing.*

Recovery might be defined as the gradual process of moving back into relationship with the larger world around you. This is similar to the developmental stages children go through as their world expands to include loyalty to and belief in their family, their friends, then their school, their community, state, country, and hopefully to the whole planet.

At the height of the cardiac crisis, your attention was necessarily focused on yourself. As you emerge, you may experience dissatisfaction, restlessness, and an urge to search your life for new meaning.

Questions about the deeper changes of your life signal the final stop on the road to recovery. They're different from the questions you've dealt with regarding changes in diet and exercise, life-style, or family concerns. Modern day ethicist, Daniel C. Maguire, suggests that just as the body needs oxygen, the mind/soul needs meaning.[1] These questions point to a new perspective, a philosophic shift, an enhanced understanding of the meaning of life that can only be gleaned from experience.

Before Reid's bypass surgery, everything in Susan's life was "perfect." A self-described optimist, Susan, a forty-year-old interior decorator and mother of two, always maintained a positive attitude, no matter what problems she confronted.

In the first few weeks following the surgery, Susan carried on with her usual buoyancy and enthusiasm, answering all queries about Reid's health with the response, "He's doing great, couldn't be better!"

One afternoon during Reid's nap, Susan was watching television when a public service announcement about heart disease came on. Suddenly Susan began to cry. Without knowing why, she felt as if her heart were breaking. As the tears flowed, Susan began to feel her disappointment, exhaustion, and fear. She was sick and tired of pretending that everything was fine. In that split second, she gave herself permission to be human.

From that moment forward, Susan's journey including heart disease also contains the potential for new and richer meaning. Another spouse expressed it like this: "I've been transformed by heart disease...if I had to go back to being the person I was before all this happened, I'd choose it again." Viktor Frankl, a World War II concentration camp survivor and twentieth-century philosopher, wrote:
Man's main concern is not to gain plesure or to avoid pain but rather to see a meaning in his life. That is why man is even ready to suffer, on the condition, to be sure, that his suffering has a meaning.[2]

Religious beliefs are also tested by the cardiac crisis. Valerie, a fifty-eight-year-old cardiac spouse, struggled with doubts. Having come to her marriage with a strong religious background, she established her family's routine to include church and regular evening prayer. She taught Sunday school and was active in church activities.

After Walter's heart attack, Valerie felt that God had abandoned her. She wrestled with the question, "If there's a God, how could He allow this to happen?" She analyzed her life, trying to understand why *she* "deserved" such bad luck. In order to avoid feeling like a hypocrite, she turned away from the God she had trusted simplistically since childhood. She resigned from her job as Sunday school teacher, and for a while stopped attending church altogether. Questioning, as a cardiac spouse, what she had accepted blindly as a child eventually led Valerie to a renewed faith and a deeper understanding of God, herself, and her world.

The cardiac crisis is an awakening. We can no longer count on all that we once took for granted. What we didn't even notice before is now revealed to be something precious.

I wouldn't have wished heart disease on Marsh, or anyone. But it certainly woke me up. Our marriage and our lives had settled into a comfortably predictable pattern. Married for over twenty years, we had long ago lost the sense of mystery and excitement that earlier had marked our relationship. We knew each other well, had learned to sidestep our differences, and over time had softened the rough edges of our relationship. We had deepened the groove by long habit and had reached a point where we took each other for granted, not the sort of atmosphere in which growth blossoms. We had reached the "flabby forties." We were settled down and settled in.

Coming to terms with the idea of a limited *quantity* of life opens the cardiac spouse to think about *quality* of life. As a result of your experience, you find yourself questioning your values, priorities, and beliefs. Your relationships with your mate, your family, and your spirituality are suddenly significant and genuine concerns.

We're often blind to changes within us. Beth, a thirty-year-old cardiac spouse, experienced what she described as a surprising need for spiritual support. In the middle of the night before her husband Gary's surgery, she awoke with a start. She was terrified and shaking. She tried telling herself that everything was all right and that Gary would make it through the operation. But she couldn't silence her fears. Beth got out of bed and walked outside where she stood alone in the darkness beneath the stars. Suddenly, she began to pray. Although Beth had never thought of herself as religious, her prayer was the comfort she needed at that moment. Opening her heart on that dark night was the beginning of a new faith for Beth. And her faith translated into a new career; Beth recently completed chaplaincy training and is working with cardiac families in a metropolitan hospital.

Beth's story illustrates how personal experience can translate into a more meaningful life, actively working to help make things better. Not everyone changes careers or makes dramatic life changes as a result of the cardiac crisis. In *Fire In The Soul*, Joan Borysenko, Ph.D. writes, "...each wound we suffer and eventually heal from is a soul-making experience with the potential to awaken our willingness to participate in the healing of the world."[3] There's only one piece of advice applicable here: Allow *your* heart to open, and let your open heart guide your life. Living from your heart can make your daily activity and your most important relationships a celebration of life.

Service is a natural human tendency.[4] Acting because you think you "should," or in order to "be good" is draining and exhausting. Service nourishes you as you give. We are spontaneously drawn to do service. It is the natural outpouring of the human heart.

> *Until I was about forty, I spent most of my energy trying to "do good" without knowing why. In retrospect, I deeply believed that I was bad; the only way to hide my shadow from others and earn their love was to be a do-gooder.*
>
> *I was sure that someone other than I knew the right way to "do good" and I was determined to learn how. I experimented with various yogas, diets, meditations, and*

therapy. I read every self-help book I could lay my hands on. I studied various psychologies, even shifted careers, leaving teaching to become a psychotherapist, hoping that by helping others, I might get fixed too.

I was a continual disappointment to myself; my feet would fall asleep as I tried to sit in the lotus position. I felt nauseated, not enlightened, by the odor of incense. I always felt like either a fraud or a failure with someone else's answers. It was like wearing the wrong pair of shoes; either they pinched because they were too tight, weren't a color that matched my clothes, or made me trip because they were too wide and fell off my feet.

One evening about a year after Marsh's bypass surgery, I accepted an invitation to a meditation service to be led by a real Tibetan lama. I arrived a few minutes late, and sat down in the back of a room filled with chanting Americans. At first I was absorbed, not by the holiness or the mystery, but by my curiosity: how many Westerners were stuffed into this room, all shoeless, many sitting in uncomfortable poses. (At my age, the posture, if I could even get into it, would mean a sore back the next day for sure.) Some were chanting in a unified response to the lama, who was draped in red and had a shaved head.

Once I got a sense of what was going on, I let myself wonder what I was doing there. I recalled the many evenings I had spent similarly, leaving my family and racing off to hear a speaker, an author, a teacher, a guru. And always I returned home disappointed, never finding the answer I had hoped for.

I started to think about what I had done in the past that had given me satisfaction. I recalled how meaningful it had been to create a hospital program for the families of dying patients in the early 1970s. I knew the need for the program, because of my experience at that hospital when my mother died.

My most recent work with cardiac spouses had come from my own heart as well. I felt great empathy for the unrecognized suffering and lack of support for cardiac spouses everywhere.

Sitting in that room, while everyone chanted, I began to understand. What is spiritual for me is participating in the human task of "making things better" when I understand the need from my own experience. I began that night to accept that I have something to offer, something to give, something that can help. I don't have to don funny clothes, assume strange postures, or eat weird foods to feel good about myself and to have a meaningful life. All I have to do is stay open, trust, and respond to the opportunities presented in my own life.

As I continue to do "my" work, I celebrate life by giving something back to the world. I have been richly blessed, and I have suffered. I no longer yearn to study one more discipline, or feel tempted to make the circuit for one more lecture.

It's still somewhat unsettling to acknowledge that I am at peace with myself, my life, my spirituality. But each time I do, I know more surely that the way of my own heart is a spiritual way. At the same time, I feel more tolerant and compassionate toward others whose journeys are different; they are searching for their unique paths and trying to understand the meaning of their lives.

I have no intention, by sharing my own story, to push or pull any cardiac spouse toward any specific course. I have been enriched by the many cardiac spouses who have shared their lives, their struggles, and their successes with me. Some of the most beautiful stories have been the most simple. Nothing could be more stirring than heartmates expressing an increased awareness of their love, their eagerness to express it, and their courage to face the reality of their lives with increased meaning and hope for the future.

I have shared my personal story throughout this book to demonstrate that although I will always be a cardiac spouse and Marsh has heart disease forever, it didn't mean an end to all that was good in our lives. I believe that out of the cardiac experience, your life can become richer, more meaningful, and more joyous. Heart disease doesn't have to be an end. It can be a new beginning.

CHAPTER NOTES

1. From a 1993 lecture presented in Minneapolis by Daniel C. Maguire, Professor of Ethics at Marquette University, author of *The Moral Core of Judaism and Christianity.*
2. From *The Doctor and The Soul*, Viktor E. Frankl, M.D. (New York: Vintage/Random House, 1955). See especially the sections on "The Meaning of Life," and "The Meaning of Suffering."
3. From *Fire In The Soul: A New Psychology of Spiritual Optimism,* Joan Borysenko, Ph.D. (New York: Warner Books, 1993). I recommend this book because it is so useful as people begin to explore spirituality.
4. See the section on "Service" in John Firman and James Vargiu's article "Dimensions of Growth," in *Synthesis* 3-4, available only in libraries. Also see Ram Dass and Paul Gorman's book, How Can I Help? (New York: Alfred A. Knopf, 1985), an elegant and touching study of the simplicity of service. People serve by moving in both directions: some of us heal ourselves by participating in healing the world, and others of us focus on healing ourselves and by doing so participate in healing the world. "Let there be peace on earth and let it begin with me."

APPENDIX A

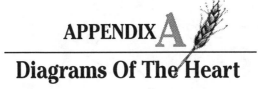

Diagrams Of The Heart

These four drawings illustrate the arterial blockages that cause heart attack and the bypass graft which can compensate for the damage caused by blocked arteries.

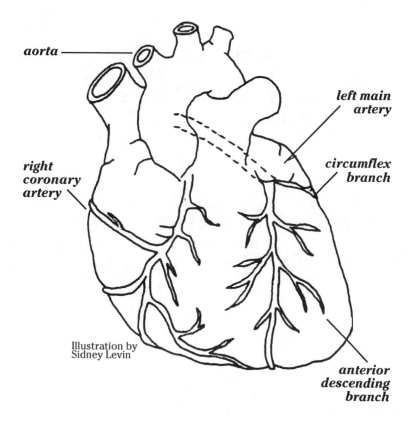

aorta

left main
artery

right
coronary
artery

circumflex
branch

Illustration by
Sidney Levin

anterior
descending
branch

The Normal Heart

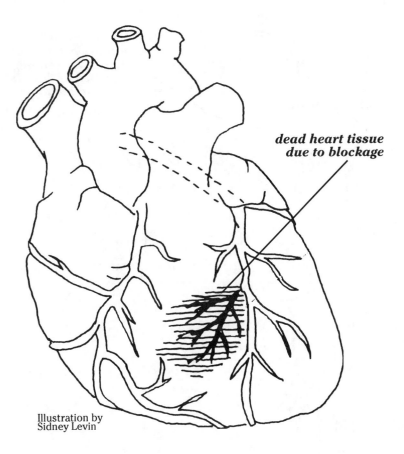

*dead heart tissue
due to blockage*

Illustration by
Sidney Levin

**Blockage
(Myocardial Infarction)**

*Partial blockage of right
coronary artery and
anterior descending
branch of the left
main artery*

Illustration by
Sidney Levin

Partially Obstructed Heart

grafts bypassing blockages

Illustration by
Sidney Levin

Double Bypass Grafts

APPENDIX B
Self-help Tools

Relaxation

Relaxing your body and mind is a crucial component of recovery. Biofeedback and meditation are practical skills to help manage the stress of the cardiac crisis. Check local community education programs or your cardiac rehabilitation program for availability of classes.

Here is a simple exercise that requires no more than ten minutes a day. It can be done at the beginning and/or end of the day; taking ten minutes in the middle of the day can be revitalizing as well. To be effective, it should be done daily, preferably at the same time and in the same place. Have someone read the exercise to you the first few times, until you can follow the order without the distraction of having to read it. Or record it for yourself on audio tape leaving enough pause time to follow each direction.

RELAXATION EXERCISE

Sit in a comfortable chair, with your spine straight and your feet flat on the floor. Close your eyes and focus your attention on your breath, following its natural cycle in and out. With each inhalation, be aware that you are taking in clean and clear energy. Experience the release of tension as you exhale. Allow your breathing to remain neutral, don't change it in any way, just notice that with each breath you are more in touch with your depth and you become more relaxed.

Focus now on your body so that it can relax and you can let go of the tension you carry there. Begin with your feet: first your right foot, then your left. Imagine all of the tension flowing out through the bottom of your feet and into the earth below. Now allow the muscles in your calves and thighs to relax as well. First your right leg, then, your left. Your legs feel warm and loose. Now pay attention to your abdomen, where you may feel tightness and stress. Let your breath flow through your abdomen, and let go of the tension. Now focus on your back, with its many muscles, and your shoulders. Breathe energy into your shoulders, and feel the tension let go. Now attend to your arms, first the right, then, the left. Let go, first in your upper arm, then the lower part, and last your hands and each of your fingers. Experience the tightness flowing out of every fingertip. Feel your neck relaxed and free as the tension flows from it. Concentrate now on your jaw, letting it relax, letting your mouth open naturally as you let go of holding it tight. Now focus on your eyes and allow them to let go. Feel the muscles behind your eyes relaxing and expanding. And last, the top and back of your head. Feel your head get light and clear as your mind stops racing. You are alert but not busy. Now that your body is relaxed, focus once again on your breath. Breathe in whatever quality you need at this moment - calm, peace, serenity, patience, freedom, compassion, love - and exhale any remaining tension or tightness.

Imagine yourself in a beautiful green meadow. You are able to rest and be nurtured by the beauty of nature surrounding you. You feel the warm sun on your skin, the solid earth holds you securely. The air is fresh and there is a pleasant cool breeze. You can smell grasses and wildflowers. You hear birds singing and the babble of a nearby brook. Take some time to enjoy the peace and the calm. Allow yourself to be filled and quieted.

Stay in this serene and beautiful place as long as you are comfortable. When you are ready, focus your attention on your breathing again. Breathe as fully and deeply as you naturally can. Notice how you feel as you do. Now, very gently, bring your awareness back to the present and slowly open your eyes. Take a moment to stretch your body as tall as you can when you rise and return to your everyday reality.

THE EVENING REVIEW

The Evening Review is a daily exercise designed to enhance personal growth. It is particularly useful to the cardiac spouse because it provides a structure to establish regular introspection, a quiet time when you can think about your day. It can help you focus on questions about life raised by the cardiac crisis. The process of doing the exercise facilitates acceptance of reality, in regular and small steps.

The Evening Review can be used as a recovery tool, helping the cardiac spouse to focus on him- or herself.

Reviewing is a mental activity, naturally operating during a crisis, that helps a person to think clearly, see reality, and establish order in the chaos of the crisis.

Evening Review Exercise

The review is best done as the last activity of your day. Before going to sleep, review your day in your mind, "playing" it like a movie, backward, beginning where you are right now, then the time of late evening, then the time of early evening, then the dinner hour, the afternoon, and so on to the morning when you awakened.

This exercise can be used to examine yourself and your life as a whole. It can be modified, as in the example below, to focus on some aspect of yourself, on some inner process or pattern you'd like to know more about. The attitude with which you do the exercise is most important. When you examine your day, do it as much as possible as the detached, objective observer, calmly and clearly registering each phase of what has happened. Then move on to the next phase without excitement, without becoming elated at a success or unhappy about a failure. The aim is to calmly register awareness of the meaning and patterns of the day, rather than to relive it.

Many have found it valuable to write down, perhaps as part of a journal or your Heartmates® diary, observations, insights, or impressions. By reviewing your notes over a period of time, you may discover patterns and trends not otherwise apparent.

REVIEW OF BOUNDARIES

This modification of the Evening Review consists of reviewing your day from the point of view of your boundaries. Psychological boundaries are protective membranes best used to deflect what is detrimental to the system and to attract what nourishes it. (Consider how skillfully a plant protects itself from poisonous or unneeded elements and finds nutrients in the appropriate quantities to sustain growth.)

Before doing this exercise the first time, you might identify activities and relationships that are particularly nourishing or depleting at this point in your life. If you keep a journal, reviewing recent writings may provide insight.

As part of your Evening Review, some of the things that you may want to keep in mind are:[1]

1. What is my experience of my boundaries? Have there been changes in my boundary system since the cardiac crisis began? Are there changes as I become aware of my boundaries and how I use them?

2. How do I evaluate environmental influences? From which can I get nourishment or from which do I need protection?

3. How skillful am I in using and shifting my boundaries? In what situations and with whom is it easy or difficult?

4. What do I allow in? What do I push away? What in myself do I protect (my heart, my mind, my body, my feelings)?

You may consider these questions during the review exercise itself, or, if this gets in your way, you may want to think about them at the end of your review. They are meant to provide a choice of perspective and all need not be covered. Their main purpose is to increase awareness of your boundaries and protection.

Keep the exercise simple, and particularly at the

beginning give it no more than fifteen minutes a day (including journal writing).

Partial Life Review

In the confusion of loss, it is the search for meaning that brings people away from dark times into the light. One of the natural ways people search is by reviewing what has happened to them in a crisis. This exercise is designed to assist cardiac spouses by structuring a way to look at a transition or loss in their past, before the cardiac crisis.

The exercise is particularly useful to find qualities and strengths already developed that have application in the present crisis. Looking at how you handled a loss or crisis in the past can familiarize you with your patterns of coping. It's likely that you will find similarities in your coping skills now. Looking at your patterns is the first step in incorporating the best of what you have done with new choices.

You may want to do the exercise more than once, focusing on other transitions you have experienced. When you are familiar with the process, you can use the exercise to look at the cardiac crisis you are experiencing in the present. Keep writing materials near; insights (like dreams) are quickly forgotten unless they are written down.

PARTIAL LIFE REVIEW EXERCISE[2]

Take a few minutes to reflect on several periods of transition or events that were turning points in your life. Begin by jotting them down on paper. They might include a major decision you made some time ago, the loss of a relationship that has affected you, or something that happened on a larger scale, outside yourself, that has had an influence on your life.

Now, from those events you have written down, choose one that you are willing to look at in a more detailed way.

First, recall the period of your life when the event happened. What was going on within you, outside you? Who were the important people in your life? Was there a person or persons that you confided in? Were you alone, without support? As you review this period of your life, see yourself as you were then.

Now recall how you acted, what kinds of things you did at the time of the event (the decision, transition, choice, loss). What was your behavioral response to the event itself?

As you see yourself in retrospect, how did you feel about what was happening to you? Notice the progression of feelings that occurred as the experience happened. Your feelings at the onset of the period may have been very different from what you felt later as you integrated the experience into your life. Notice, too, whether you expressed your feelings directly then, or whether you pushed them down or away. Did you express some feelings and suppress others? As you look back, can you see any of your feelings being expressed indirectly? Did anyone important to you know how you were feeling then?

Shift your focus of attention to your thoughts at the time of the event. What were you aware of, considering, weighing, judging? Notice whether you did that thinking alone or whether there was someone you discussed those thoughts with. At that time did you think that what was happening was an opportunity? Did it make sense to you in the larger context of your life?

Now, bring yourself and your awareness back to

the present, being aware that whatever the event was, you are beyond it now. With the passage of time, and reviewing it now, does the event make sense in relation to your life? Is there something you can see about it now that you couldn't see then? Does reviewing this particular event change how you see yourself, your image? Are you now more understanding, judgmental, compassionate, accepting, forgiving of what you did, how you felt, or what you thought of yourself then? Is there anything you learned then (a skill or a quality that was developed) that can be useful to you in your life now?

Is there anything in this review that points toward your future . . . any new way you'd like to act or live, think, or feel, having looked clearly at the past? What are the implications for the future, now that you have reviewed the past in this way?

When you have finished looking, take time to write about what you've learned. If it makes sense to continue the process, you may want to share your review with someone important in your life. You may want to focus on this event, its implications, and the pattern(s) revealed in a regular Evening Review for a period of time.

Family Meeting: Problem-solving Model

When difficult decisions need to be made and long-term changes need to be accepted and integrated, families may feel vulnerable and unprepared. Old conflicts may erupt to complicate the present issues. New roles and evolving family rules may need to be clarified. Establishing regular family council meetings to discuss problems and seek solutions is one way to deal with the cardiac crisis as a family.

Family council meetings should be scheduled for a definite day and time, weekly. Each meeting should be led by a different member of the family. The responsibility of record-keeping (in summary or "minutes" form) should also be shared. Meetings should be no longer than one hour. Family members of all ages should be included, if possible. I recommend that children as young as elementary school age attend. They will learn from being included, even if they have little to contribute at first. The family will experience success if all members are willing to approach issues as family problems. The solution to problems is as much a family responsibility as are the problems. This approach develops mutual respect and cooperation and promotes family support and cohesion.

Here is a six-step guide your family can follow to solve problems together.

1. Together make a list of all the family concerns. Anything unresolved in the eyes of one family member belongs on the list. Be wary of commenting on contributions. This is not the place or the time to share feelings about any one problem. Don't permit anyone to blame anyone else for any problem. The purpose of this family activity is to seek solutions to the dilemmas of the family.

2. Together, select the three to five most critical issues. Selection should take into account which issues are the most pressing and which are the most important. The remainder of the list should be deferred for discussion at a later time.

3. Together, define what information is needed and which family members are responsible for data collection. The goal of this step in the problem-solving process is to gather all the ideas, information, and outside resources that will help the family to resolve the issues.

Individual family members should also reflect on their own ideas about each of the critical problems during this period of time.

4. Meet together to share information and resources. The purpose of this meeting is to share all the information and ideas on each of the critical issues to be resolved. Respect for each person's ideas and attentive listening to the data gathered are essential for success at this step.

5. Share individual ideas for solutions/resolutions. Every solution offered by family members should be heard and considered. One family member can be designated as secretary for each issue, responsible for putting each solution in writing. The most pressing problem should be discussed first, followed by the others in the priority of their importance.

6. Together, agree on a best solution. By consensus, negotiation, and compromise, the family agrees to a resolution. The family also needs to decide what actions will accomplish resolution, and what each family member needs to do. Before a next set of issues is taken on by the family, there should be a follow-up meeting to assure that resolution on issues being worked on is complete. Celebrate each solution as a family!

APPENDIX B NOTES:

1. Adapted from the unpublished writings of Roberto Assagioli.
2. Adapted from Rhoda F. Levin, "Life Review: A Natural

Process," in *Readings in Psychosynthesis: Theory, Process, and Practice* (Toronto: Ontario Institute for Studies in Education, 1985), p. 96.

APPENDIX C

Heartmates® Recommended Reading List

Companion Through the Darkness: Inner Dialogues on Grief. Stephanie Ericsson, New York: HarperCollins, 1993.

The Dance of Anger: A Woman's Guide to Changing the Patterns of Intimate Relationships. Harriet Goldhor Lerner, Ph.D., New York: Harper & Row, 1986.

The Dance of Intimacy: A Woman's Guide to Courageous Acts of Change in Key Relationships. Harriet Goldhor Lerner, Ph.D., New York: Harper & Row, 1989.

Fire In The Soul: A New Psychology of Spiritual Optimism. Joan Borysenko, New York: Warner Books, 1993.

The Healing Heart. Norman Cousins, New York: W.W. Norton & Co., 1983.

Heart Illness and Intimacy, How Caring Relationships Aid Recovery. Wayne M. Sotile, Ph.D., Baltimore: The Johns Hopkins University Press, 1992.

Kinds of Loss. Alla Renée Bozarth, Ph.D., Minneapolis, MN.: Compcare Publications, 1982.

Learned Optimism. Martin E.P. Seligman, Ph.D., New York: Alfred A. Knopf, Inc., 1990.

Life's Companion: Journal Writing As a Spiritual Quest. Christina Baldwin, New York: Bantam Books, 1990.

Love, Medicine & Miracles. Bernie S. Siegel, M.D., New York: Harper & Row, 1986.

Mainstay: For the Well Spouse of the Chronically Ill. Maggie Strong, Boston: Little, Brown & Co., 1988.

Men Are from Mars, Women Are from Venus: A Practical Guide for Improving Communication and Getting What You Want in Your Relationships. John Gray, Ph.D., New York: HarperCollins, 1992.

Necessary Losses. Judith Viorst, New York: Simon & Schuster, 1986.

The Right to Feel Bad. Lesley Hazelton, New York: Random House, 1984.

Sailing. Susan Kenney, New York: Viking Penguin Inc., 1988, a novel about a middle-aged woman whose husband has cancer.

Stones for Ibarra. Harriet Doerr, New York: Penguin Books, 1978, a beautiful first novel by an elderly woman about a couple struggling with life-threatening illness.

Soul Mates: Honoring the Mysteries of Love and Relationship. Thomas Moore, New York: HarperCollins, 1994.

Two-Part Invention, The Story of a Marriage. Madeleine L'Engle, New York: Farrar, Straus & Giroux, 1988, an autobiography about the love of two very independent people in the last years of one of their lives.

When Bad Things Happen to Good People. Rabbi Harold S. Kushner, New York: Schocken Books, Inc., 1981.

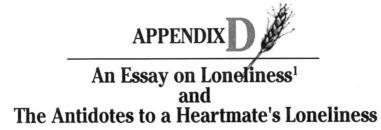

APPENDIX D

An Essay on Loneliness[1]
and
The Antidotes to a Heartmate's Loneliness

Over the years since I first wrote *Heartmates®* I have received many letters describing the loneliness of life as a heartmate. One of the most poignant was from a forty-five-year-old California woman, who wrote:

"My spouse [the heart patient] has read *Heartmates®* too and feels greater understanding about the issues his illness has raised for me, for us, and the family. *Heartmates®* allowed him to **step aside for a moment from his role as patient and be my friend again.** It's been a hard and tender time of deep change."

The question arises: How is it that what we want most, **to feel loved and understood by our mates,** is so difficult, so out of our reach, so impossible to grasp? The fact of heart disease provides real and legitimate reasons for the loneliness of the heartmate.

1. Heartmates are given a strong message in the hospital (by our limited access to our mate and by the hush-hush atmosphere maintained in the coronary care unit) that the pa-

tient must be protected from stress. How we interpret the message, in our shock and terror, is that we - our presence and our very being - are dangerous to the patient. We could cause another cardiac event, even our loved one's death, if we don't learn to behave appropriately.

2. Many heartmates believe that expressing feelings and thoughts may be contagious. Early in recovery we begin to set aside or "push away" our negative thoughts and feelings believing that we are protecting the patient and the rest of the family. We want to make sure they are not "brought down" by the way we feel. Natural feelings, like fear, sadness, disappointment, depression, and resentment, as well as realistic and practical concerns, become unacceptable topics for discussion.

3. Family and friends expect heartmates to express gratitude for the patient's survival. Professional caregivers expect a heartmate to be a consistent cheerleader for the patient. Outsiders think that just because our mates have survived and are physically recovering everything has returned to normal. Non-heartmates don't understand (because they've not had the experience) that the heartmate's life has permanently changed. They don't know we have losses to grieve and adjustments to make in order to come to terms with our new reality. They don't realize that there is no going back to a pre-heart disease normal.

4. Heart patients are wrapped up in their own health and recovery. They are the center of attention from concerned others. Their physical and psychic energies are being consumed with their own healing and their serious concerns about their own survival. They don't have energy available to pay attention to the needs of others. Of course, for the heartmate, this can be the deepest source of loneliness.

So heartmates live in an atmosphere in which loneliness

seems inevitable. Neither our mates, family and friends, not even professionals understand what is happening to us and how we feel.

But loneliness is *not* inevitable. To really understand that your experience is normal with a cardiac crisis takes hard-won self-acceptance. It takes guts to break through the wall of isolation separating you from others who have not understood you. It takes real courage to risk rebuilding the heartmate relationship, to commit to caring again, when you might lose your love.

But when we say to ourselves, "this is too hard," "it isn't worth the struggle," or "I can't do it," we must not give in. We are strong, resilient, and courageous. Look at what we have lived through already. We have found in ourselves qualities we never knew we had - strength, resiliency, indefatigability, perseverance, courage and caring - and have survived. Surely, we won't let loneliness beat us!

What's different about dealing with our own loneliness is that we have used our skills and strengths to give to others - to our recovering mates and to our families. And now it is time to ask for and receive what we ourselves need - to be heard, to be understood, to be accepted, and to be loved.

The antidotes to loneliness - steps to healing - are simple but not easy.

1. We need to accept our own thoughts and feelings. They are legitimate, okay, natural, human.

2. We need to seek support from others: those people who can hear us without trying to fix us, because we aren't broken; those people who can accept what they hear as our thoughts and feelings even if they are different from their own; those people who can listen empathetically, who can understand and feel compassion for us.

3. We need to express our thoughts and feelings with these people we have found. We need to heal our wounds by telling our stories, saying how we felt and feel, expressing our concerns.

Accepting our own thoughts and feelings and sharing them with others leads us to a new place, a place where we are no longer lonely. Simultaneously we will know our uniqueness and be connected. We will experience our aloneness and our togetherness. We will have our own place in the universe and belong with all other humans on our planet. And we will have healed ourselves from and stepped beyond a significant wound of the cardiac crisis.

Stay connected.[2] If you want to network with another heartmate through letters, we'll try to put you in touch. If you have questions, thoughts or feelings you want to share, call The Heartmates® Heartline at (612) 929-3331, fax us at (612) 929-6395, contact us at our electronic mail address: heartmates@aol.com or write us at:

The Heartmates® Connection
Box 16202
Minneapolis, MN 55416

APPENDIX D NOTES:

1. The original draft of this essay was for a magazine for heart patients and spouses, called *HeartCorps*, which failed after a couple of years because of insufficient subscriptions. Although several Heartmates® essays were printed there, the most important one, on Loneliness, has been in my computer until this revision.

2. Because of the isolation of cardiac spouses, I tried to do a

national newsletter, which I called *The Heartmates® Connection*. After only three issues I found I couldn't do it all myself, and at that time I was producing the videoseries of five programs called *Portrait of a Heartmate*. I still believe strongly that connection, listening, telling our stories, is what can heal us individually and can help build human community. Perhaps time and technology are now on our side, and through E-Mail and mail, phone and fax, *The Heartmates® Connection* can function as it was originally intended, to provide support and community to an undeservedly isolated population.

APPENDIX E

An Essay on Stress: Living with and Controlling Stress

Stress can be defined as any response of the body to demands placed on it. Stress can be both positive and negative. The demands require the body to make some adjustment in order to reestablish harmony. When the demand is made, adrenaline and cortisol are released and your body responds by going into the "fight or flight" syndrome. When you need the extra strength or stamina to fight or flee, your body responds because of the adrenaline.

Stress exists both inside and outside of us. It affects us before birth and until we die. It affects us socially, spiritually, emotionally, and psychologically. The link between stress and illness is not so much the illness, but our response to that illness. In other words, having a spouse with heart disease will cause heartmates to respond differently. This can also be true for any external situation that causes stress. Moments of stress followed by a physical reaction are not necessarily harmful. But when psychological response to stress is not discharged, it accumulates, causing chronic stress. This can produce hormonal imbalances and is a setup for disease - it puts us at risk.

Dis-ease means the body is not at ease. Prolonged stress affects our bodies at their weakest points. Tension headaches, backaches, migraines, stomach pains, anxiety, ulcers, and changes in the immune system have all been linked to prolonged stress.

Stress can be beneficial. A certain amount of stress helps us to concentrate, stay focused, perform, and even achieve peak efficiency. Many people perform well under stress. The key is to relax and enjoy the achievements. This enables the body to build for the next challenge.

Stress can be an attempt of the body to heal itself. When a situation, relationship, or illness is causing stress, the person may be forced to look at what is causing the stress and make changes. Changes in behavior or changing an emotional response may be healing.

Stress management then implies two things:
1. Stress is inevitable.
2. We can use stress to change our lives.

The key to stress management is awareness. Know what your stressors are, and how stress affects you. **Discover your feelings** (emotions) and learn to deal with them in a healthy way. Develop positive mental attitudes and turn them into positive actions. Learn what problem-solving skills you have, and which ones you need to improve on.

When stress becomes dis-stress, **get support** from friends, family, support groups.

Practice a regular exercise program. This keeps your body in balance, increases stamina, and decreases your appetite. Maintain a healthy diet. Drink eight glasses of water a day. This also keeps your body in physical balance.

Engage in relaxation exercises, meditation, massage, yoga, or biofeedback. Any one of these will help calm your body, and therefore your mind.

Develop spiritually! By doing so, you will find that you are never alone, and you have someone or thing with whom to ease your burden.

Maintain a positive self-image. Recognize your needs and make positive choices to support those needs. Learn to let go of situations beyond your control, and remember, there are very few situations or people we actually control.

Learn to laugh - at yourself and with others. Studies have shown that laughter increases the immune response of the body. Always maintain a sense of hope. And last, but not least, live in the present and look forward to the future.

This article was contributed by Pamela R. Borgmann, RN, M.Th. Her current career includes massage therapy and health education. She lives with her husband and two children in Minneapolis, Minnesota.

GLOSSARY
Medical Terms

Aneurysm. A weakness in an artery or vein in the wall of your heart muscle that forms a balloonlike bulge.

Angina. The heart muscle's complaint that it is not receiving enough blood or oxygen. It frequently occurs when the heart works harder than usual, such as during exercise, stress, sexual intercourse, walking in extremely hot or cold weather, or after eating a large meal. Anginal discomfort can be experienced in a variety of ways. It can feel like chest pain, pressure, or heaviness. It can feel like a pain or ache in the jaw, teeth, or earlobes, or be a choking or tightening sensation in the throat. It can be experienced as pain, aching, or numbness in one or both arms or hands, between the shoulder blades, or in the neck. Anginal discomfort may start in one place and move to another (i.e., chest pain that spreads to the shoulder and down the arm). It is important to know that angina is not just felt as "chest pain," but as a variety of symptoms. Angina is usually brief (from thirty seconds to five minutes) and may disappear slowly or quickly. Angina is not a heart attack.

Angiogram. An X-ray picture of the coronary arteries. In the procedure, a catheter (specialized tube) is inserted into an artery in the groin. It follows the artery's path up to the heart, where, through the tube, dye is injected while filming is done. These films show areas of narrowing or blockage in the coronary arteries and help the cardiologist and cardiac surgeon plan the most effective treatment. This procedure takes about an hour and has some risk involved, but it is the most precise reading of coronary artery blockage available. After the procedure, the patient must lie flat for a number of hours to prevent the artery from reopening and bleeding.

Angioplasty. (See Balloon angioplasty)

Aorta. The large main artery that leaves the heart delivering freshly oxygenated blood to all parts of the body.

Arrhythmia. Any change in the normal rhythm of the heart.

Arteries. These are the blood vessels that carry fresh (oxygenated) blood from the heart to all parts of the body. (Veins are the blood vessels that bring used blood back to the heart.)

Arteriosclerosis. A progressive condition that causes the artery walls to thicken and lose their elasticity. Also called "hardening of the arteries."

Atherosclerosis. This is a form of arteriosclerosis, in which the passageways through the arteries become roughened and narrowed by fatty deposits (see Plaque) that harden along the inner lining of the arteries.

Balloon angioplasty. A procedure used to open clogged arteries. A special balloon catheter (tube) is inserted into an artery in the groin, as in the angiogram procedure. The catheter is positioned into the narrowed portion of the coronary artery, and the balloon is inflated. The balloon compresses the plaque, widening the narrowed area of the passageway, to increase the flow of blood and oxygen to the heart muscle.

Bypass surgery (also referred to as coronary artery bypass surgery, CAB, CABS). This operation uses a blood vessel from another part of the body to bypass the blocked area in the coronary artery (see diagram). A clean blood vessel is sewn above and below the blockage in the coronary artery. It is the construction of a new pathway for blood to flow around the narrowed section of artery to the heart muscle. Picture the surgery as providing a detour around a traffic jam, so that cars can get where they're going unimpeded. The procedure should improve the blood flow to the heart muscle. Angina is relieved for 90 percent of those who have bypass surgery.

Blood enzyme test. Cardiac enzymes are substances that are normally stored in the heart muscle. During an injury to the heart (i.e., a heart attack), these enzymes are released into the bloodstream. Several blood samples are drawn after a suspected heart attack to check for these enzymes. This blood test helps to determine whether or not a heart attack has occurred. It usually takes twenty-four to forty-eight hours after the suspected heart attack to get results.

Blood pressure. The pressure placed on the walls of your arteries as your heart pumps blood. The top number (systolic) refers to the pressure in your arteries while your heart is contracting, and the bottom number (diastolic) refers to the pressure in your arteries when your heart is relaxed (in between beats). Hypertension is high blood pressure, usually greater than 140 over 90 in adults.

Cardiac risk factors. These are living habits, physical attributes, and characteristics or inherited tendencies that may increase the chance of developing heart disease. Risk factors include: smoking, high blood pressure, high blood cholesterol, inactivity, obesity, diabetes, stress, and heredity.

Cholesterol. A fat-like substance found only in animal products (highest in organ meats), dairy products, and eggs. The cholesterol present in our blood stream originates from the cholesterol we eat plus what we produce ourselves. Elevated blood cholesterol is associated with an increased risk of atherosclerosis. Cholesterol can be broken down (see Lipoproteins).

Congestive heart failure. A condition in which a weakened heart is not able to adequately pump the blood around the body. Poor circulation results, and fluid may collect in the lungs, ankles, and feet.

Coronary arteries. Three main arteries and their branches (see diagram), that supply the heart muscle with blood, oxygen, and nutrients. If these arteries become narrowed by atherosclerosis, angina or a heart attack can occur.

CPR (Cardiopulmonary resuscitation). A lifesaving skill, often called mouth-to-mouth resuscitation, that is taught by the American Red Cross. I recommend that all cardiac spouses become certified in CPR. Preparation and training may help you save a life. You will also gain confidence in your ability to respond appropriately and efficiently in an emergency.

Echocardiogram. A way of viewing the heart without entering the body. This technique uses high frequency sound waves for measuring and determining the function and structure of the heart. It is completely painless and takes from one half to one hour to complete. Echocardiograms cannot see coronary arteries at this time, and therefore cannot be used to pinpoint the narrowed arteries (see Angiogram).

EKG (Electrocardiogram). A recording of the electrical currents produced by the heart. These electrical currents are responsible for the beating of the heart muscle. A resting EKG can detect any abnormal beats and can determine if the heart muscle is presently not receiving enough blood and oxygen, or if heart damage was done in the past. It is a painless procedure of attaching suction cups to the skin.

Endotracheal tube. A tube placed in the windpipe through which air and oxygen are passed to aid breathing, used in surgery or with very ill patients. Bypass patients complain about the frustration of this tube because they can't speak. Having a pad and pencil, small chalkboard, or "magic slate" available can enhance the patient's ability to communicate until the tube is removed (usually twenty-four to forty-eight hours after surgery).

Exercise. Forms of physical activity done by cardiac patients for the purposes of reducing risk factors, increasing physical fitness, and possibly improving cardiac function and the quality of life. The activities that seem to produce these results are walking, jogging, bicycling, swimming, and rowing (aerobic exercises). It is generally recommended that individuals with heart disease engage in these activities three to five times a week for a twenty- to forty-five-minute session. Check with your personal physician for more specific guidelines.

Heart attack (also called a myocardial infarction, an MI, or a coronary thrombosis). This occurs when the flow of blood to a part of the heart muscle is suddenly cut off or severely diminished. A part of the heart muscle dies in a heart attack (See diagram).

Lipoproteins (HDL, LDL). Fats carried in the blood, also known as "good cholesterol" (HDL) and "bad cholesterol" (LDL). Abnormal levels of these fats are associated with heart and blood vessel disease.Triglycerides are another type of fat found in the bloodstream; a modest elevation of triglycerides is probably not an important risk factor for heart disease, unless the blood cholesterol is also elevated. High triglyceride levels are found more commonly in overweight and/or diabetic individuals, who consume a high-fat diet.

MEDICATIONS:

Anticoagulants. (Also referred to incorrectly as "blood thinners," they do not actually thin the blood.) These medications are used to improve the flow of blood and prevent the formation of blood clots. (Blood clots blocking the coronary arteries can cause a heart attack.)

Antiarrhythmics. These are a group of medications that regulate irregular heart rhythms.

Antihypertensives. Medications of many types, used to lower high blood pressure.

Beta-blockers. A group of medications used to treat high blood pressure. Some beta-blockers are used to help relieve angina, and are taken to help prevent additional heart attacks. One side effect of beta-blockers is reduced libido or impotency. Often switching to a different beta-blocker will eliminate the side effect.

Calcium channel blockers. A group of medications used to treat angina by increasing the supply of blood and oxygen to the heart while reducing the work of the heart.

Cholesterol reducers. Medication that lowers the level of cholesterol in the blood.

Diuretics. Medications that increase the output of urine, therefore helping to reduce the amount of fluid and sodium in the body. They can be used to treat high blood pressure and congestive heart failure.

Nitrates. Medication commonly prescribed to treat angina. They work by increasing the supply of blood and oxygen to the heart, while reducing the work of the heart. They may be prescribed in several forms: a tablet to be dissolved under the tongue, a tablet to be swallowed, an ointment or a patch to be applied to the skin.

Nitroglycerin. A commonly prescribed fast-acting medication used to treat angina (see Nitrates).
Vasodilators. A group of medications that dilate blood vessels, which increases the blood flow to that area.

Pacemaker. A mechanical implant that stimulates and

regulates the heartbeat by a series of regular electrical discharges.

Plaque. In heart disease, this refers to a patchy deposit of fatty material consisting of cholesterol, calcium, and other materials, found on the inner lining of the coronary arteries.

Post cardiotomy syndrome (or "post myocardial infarction syndrome"or "Dressler's syndrome"). A condition of inflammation in the sac covering the heart, occurring after a heart attack or heart surgery. It is characterized by fever and chest pain (different from angina or incision pain). It is treatable with anti-inflammatory medications such as aspirin or cortisone.

Saturated fat. A type of fat usually solid at room temperature. Common sources include animal products (butter, chicken skin, marbled meats) and some vegetable products (coconut oil, palm oil, cocoa butter, and hydrogenated vegetable oils). High dietary intake of saturated fat tends to elevate the level of cholesterol in the blood. Limiting foods high in saturated fats helps to lower blood cholesterol. The U.S. Senate's Select Committee on Nutrition and Human Needs suggested in the 1980s reducing the intake of dietary fat to 30 percent of diet, and reducing cholesterol intake to 300 milligrams daily. By the mid 1990s common wisdom limits the intake of fat for a heart-healthy diet to between 10 and 25% of caloric intake.

Sodium. A mineral, most commonly found in table salt. Sodium retains fluid in the body, which can increase the work of the heart and increase blood pressure. It is usually recommended that individuals with high blood pressure or heart disease restrict the amount of sodium in their diets. There are high levels of sodium in prepared and frozen foods. Two thousand milligrams daily is a sensible level to try to maintain.

Streptokinase or t-PA. A thrombolytic drug, enzyme (or substance), that can dissolve blood clots. To be most effective, it should be administered within one hour of onset of symptoms or within thirty minutes after arriving at an emergency room. If given immediately after a heart attack begins, it can help prevent heart muscle damage and reduce mortality by dissolving blockages in the arteries and restoring coronary artery flow.

Stress test (Also called a graded exercise test, or a GXT). This procedure tests how well the heart delivers oxygenated blood during physical exertion. It is done for several purposes: It can help determine the level of fitness, be used for prescribing safe exercise levels, and/or determine the presence of heart disease. There is no such thing as passing or failing the stress test. With a doctor present, the person having a stress test is attached to an EKG machine and begins walking on a treadmill. The treadmill is started at a slow speed and elevation, and both are gradually increased. Blood pressure and EKG are monitored closely for changes in blood pressure and/or heartbeats.

Unsaturated fat. Includes polyunsaturated and monounsaturated fats, both of which help to lower the level of cholesterol in the blood. Major sources of polyunsaturated fat include liquid vegetable oils such as corn, sunflower, cottonseed, safflower, and soybean oil. Polyunsaturated fats tend to lower blood cholesterol. Monounsaturated fats are found in peanuts, peanut oil, olives, and olive oil. The general recommendation is to limit total fat intake to 30 percent of the total calories, one-third from each of the three types of fat: polyunsaturated, monounsaturated, and saturated fat.

BIBLIOGRAPHY

Achterberg, Jeanne. *Imagery in Healing*. Boston: New Science Library, 1985.

Alexander, Jo, Debi Berrow, Lisa Domitrovich, Margarita Donnelly, and Cheryl McLean, eds. *Women and Aging*. Corvalis, OR: Calyx Books, 1986.

Angelou, Maya. *On The Pulse of Morning*. New York: Random House, 1993.

Assagioli, Roberto. *The Act of Will*. New York: Viking Press, 1973.

_____. *Psychosynthesis: A Manual of Principles and Techniques*. New York: Penguin Books, 1965.

Baldwin, Christina. *Life's Companion: Journal Writing As a Spiritual Quest*. New York: Bantam Books, 1990.

Bolen, Jean Shinoda, M.D. *Goddesses in Every Woman*. New York: Harper & Row, 1984.

_____. *The Tao of Psychology, Synchronicity and the Self*. San Francisco: Harper & Row, 1979.

Borysenko, Joan, Ph.D., *Fire In The Soul: A New Psychology of Spiritual Optimism*. New York: Warner Books, 1993.

Boston Women's Health Book Collective. *Our Bodies, Ourselves*. New York: Simon & Schuster, 1971.

Bowman, Ted, M.S.W. *Loss of Dreams: A Special Kind of Grief*, 2111 Knapp Street, St. Paul, MN 55108, phone or fax: (612) 645-6058.

Bozarth-Campbell, Alla. *Life is Good-bye, Life is Hello: Grieving Well Through All Kinds of Loss*. Minneapolis: Compcare Publications, 1982.

Brecher, Edward. *Love, Sex and Aging*. Boston: Little, Brown & Co., 1984.

Bridges, William. *Transitions, Making Sense of Life's Changes.* Reading, Mass: Addison-Wesley Publishing Co., 1980.

Budnick, Herbert N., Ph.D. with Scott Robert Hays. *Heart to Heart, A Guide to the Psychological Aspects of Heart Disease.* Santa Fe: HealthPress, 1991.

Cousins, Norman. *Anatomy of an Illness.* New York: W.W. Norton & Co., 1979.

_____. *Head First: The Biology of Hope*. New York: E.P. Dutton, 1989.

_____. *The Healing Heart.* New York: W.W. Norton & Co., 1983.

Craven, Margaret. *I Heard the Owl Call My Name.* Garden City, NY: Doubleday, 1973.

Davidson, Glen W. *Understanding Mourning: A Guide for Those Who Grieve.* Minneapolis: Augsburg Press, 1984.

Doerr, Harriet. *Stones for Ibarra.* New York: Penguin Books, 1978.

Doherty, William J. & Thomas Campbell. *Families and Health.* Newbury Park, CA: Sage, 1988.

Doress, Paula Brown, Diana Laskin Siegal & The Midlife and Older Women Book Project. *Ourselves, Growing Older.* New York: Simon & Schuster, 1987.

Dreikurs, Rudolf, M.D., and Vicki Soltz. *Children: The Challenge.* New York: Hawthorn Books, 1964.

Eliot, Robert, M.D. *Stress and the Major Cardiovascular Disorders.* Mt. Kisco, NY: Futura Publishing Co., 1979.

Ericsson, Stephanie, *Companion Through the Darkness: Inner Dialogues on Grief.* New York: HarperCollins, 1993.

Ferrucci, Piero. Inevitable Grace. Los Angeles: J.P. Tarcher, 1990.

_____. *What We May Be.* Los Angeles: J.P. Tarcher, 1982.

Firman, John, and James Vargiu. "Dimensions of Growth," in *Synthesis 3-4.* Redwood City, CA: Synthesis Press, 1977.

Fossum, Merle A. and Marilyn J. Mason. *Facing Shame: Families in Recovery.* New York: W.W. Norton & Co., 1986.

Fowler, James W. *Stages of Faith.* San Francisco: Harper & Row, 1981.

Friedman, Meyer, M.D., and Ray H. Rosenman, M.D. *Type A Behavior and Your Heart.* New York: Fawcett Publications, 1974.

Gilligan, Carol. *In a Different Voice.* Cambridge, Mass: Harvard University Press, 1982.

Gray, John, Ph.D. *Men Are from Mars, Women Are from Venus: A Practical Guide for Improving Communication and Getting What You Want in Your Relationships.* New York: HarperCollins, 1992.

Halperin, Jonathan L., M.D., and Richard Levine. *Bypass.* New York: Times Books, 1985.

Hazleton, Lesley. *The Right to Feel Bad.* New York: Ballantine Books, 1984.

Hoffman, Nancy Yanes. *Change of Heart: The Bypass Experience.* New York: Harcourt Brace Jovanovich, 1985.

John-Roger & Peter McWilliams. *You Can't Afford the Luxury of a Negative Thought.* Los Angeles: Prelude Press, 1988.

Jung, Carl. *Memories, Dreams, Reflections.* New York: Vintage Books, 1965.

Kavanaugh, Robert E. *Facing Death.* Baltimore: Penguin Books, 1972.

Kenney, Susan. *Sailing.* New York: Viking Penguin Inc., 1988.

Kopp, Sheldon. *Raise Your Right Hand Against Fear, Extend the Other in Compassion.* New York: Ballantine Books, 1988.

Kübler-Ross, Elisabeth, M.D. *On Death and Dying.* New York: Macmillan Co., 1969.

Kushner, Harold S. *When All You've Ever Wanted Isn't Enough: The Search for a Life That Matters.* New York: Simon & Schuster, 1986.

_____. *When Bad Things Happen to Good People.* New York: Schocken Books, 1981.

Larsen, Earnie. *Stage II Recovery: Life Beyond Addiction.* Minneapolis: Winston Press, 1965.

Laurence, Margaret. *The Stone Angel.* Toronto: McClelland & Stewart, 1964.

Lear, Martha Weinman. *Heartsounds.* New York: Simon & Schuster, 1980.

L'Engle, Madeleine. *Two-Part Invention, The Story of a Marriage.* New York: Farrar, Straus & Giroux, 1988.

Leonard, Linda Scheirse. *The Wounded Woman.* Boulder, CO: Shambhala, 1983.

Lerner, Harriet Goldhor, Ph.D. *The Dance of Anger: A Woman's Guide to Changing the Patterns of Intimate Relationships.* New York: Harper & Row, 1986.

_____. *The Dance of Intimacy: A Woman's Guide to Courageous Acts of Change in Key Relationships.* New York: Harper & Row, 1989.

Lessing, Doris. *The Summer Before the Dark.* New York: Vintage Books, 1973.

Levin, Rhoda F. "Life Review: A Natural Process," in *Readings in Psychosynthesis: Theory, Process, and Practice.* Toronto: Ontario Institute for Studies in Education, 1985.

Lewis, C.S. *A Grief Observed.* New York: Bantam Books, 1961.

_____. *The Four Loves.* New York: Harcourt, Brace, Jovanovich, 1960.

Lifton, Robert J. and Eric Olson. *Living and Dying.* New York: Bantam Books, 1984.

Lindemann, Erich, M.D. *Beyond Grief: Studies in Crisis Intervention.* New York: Jason Aronson, Inc., 1979.

Lynch, James J. *The Broken Heart: The Medical Consequences of Loneliness.* New York: Basic Books, 1977.

Maslow, Abraham H. *The Farther Reaches of Human Nature.* New York: Penguin Books, 1971.

McDaniel, Susan H., Jeri Hepworth, William J. Doherty. *Medical Family Therapy.* New York: BasicBooks, 1992.

Miller, Alice. *Thou Shalt Not Be Aware.* New York: New American Library, 1984.

Mitchell, Kenneth R. & Herbert Anderson. *All Our Losses/All Our Griefs.* Philadelphia: The Westminster Press, 1983.

Moustakas, Clark E. *Loneliness and Love.* Englewood Cliffs, N.J: Prentice-Hall, Inc., 1972.

Napier, Augustus Y., Ph.D., and Carl A. Whitaker, M.D. *The Family Crucible.* New York: Bantam Books, 1978.

Needleman, Jacob. *The Heart of Philosophy.* New York: Bantam Books, 1982.

_____. *A Sense of the Cosmos.* New York: E.P. Dutton & CO., 1975.

Ornish, Dean, M.D. *Eat More, Weigh Less.* New York: HarperCollins, 1993.

_____. *Program for Reversing Heart Disease.* New York: Random House, 1990.

_____. *Stress, Diet, & Your Heart.* New York: Holt, Rinehart & Winston, 1982.

Peck, M. Scott, M.D. *The Road Less Traveled.* New York: Simon & Schuster, 1978.

Peele, Stanton. *Love and Addiction.* New York: New American Library, 1975.

Pincus, Lily. *Death and the Family.* New York: Random House, 1974.

Ram Dass and Paul Gorman. *How Can I Help?* New York: Alfred A. Knopf, 1985.

Rogers, Natalie. *Emerging Woman: A Decade of Midlife Transitions.* Point Reyes, CA: Personal Press, 1980.

Rubin, Lillian. *Intimate Strangers: Men and Women Together.* New York: Harper & Row, 1983.

_____. *Women of a Certain Age.* New York: Harper & Row, 1979.

Rubin, Theodore Isaac, M.D. The Angry Book. New York: Macmillan Co., 1969.

Sarton, May. *Kinds of Love.* New York: W.W. Norton & Co., 1970.

Scarf, Maggie. *Intimate Partners: Patterns in Love and Marriage.* New York: Random House, 1987.

Scott-Maxwell, Florida. *The Measure of My Days.* New York: Penguin Books, 1979.

Seligman, Martin E.P., Ph.D. *Learned Optimism.* New York: Alfred A. Knopf, Inc., 1990.

Selye, Hans, M.D. *The Stress of Life.* New York: McGraw-Hill Book Co., 1956.

Sheehy, Gail. *Passages.* New York: E.P. Dutton & Co., 1976.

Shneidman, Edwin S. *Deaths of Man.* Baltimore: Penguin Books, 1973.

Simonton, O.C., S. Simonton, and J. Creighton. *Getting Well Again.* Los Angeles: J.P. Tarcher, 1978.

Smedes, Lewis B. *Forgive and Forget: Healing the Hurts We Don't Deserve.* San Francisco: Harper & Row, 1984.

Sotile, Wayne M., Ph.D. *Heart Illness and Intimacy, How Caring Relationships Aid Recovery.* Baltimore: The Johns Hopkins University Press, 1992.

Speedling, Edward J. *Heart Attack: The Family Response at Home and in the Hospital.* New York: Tavistock Publications, 1982.

Stauffer, Edith R., Ph.D. *Unconditional Love and Forgiveness.* Burbank, CA: Triangle Publishers, 1987.

Stern, Ellen Sue. *Expecting Change.* New York: Poseidon Press, 1986.

Strommen, Merton P. & A. Irene. *Five Cries of Grief.* San Francisco: Harper San Francisco, 1993.

Strong, Maggie. *Mainstay: For the Well Spouse of the Chronically Ill.* Boston: Little, Brown & Co., 1988.

Tatelbaum, Judy. *The Courage to Grieve.* New York: Perennial Library, Harper & Row, 1980.

Veninga, Robert. *A Gift of Hope: How We Survive Our Tragedies.* Boston: Little, Brown & Co., 1985.

Viorst, Judith. *Necessary Losses.* New York: Fawcett Gold Medal, 1986.

Waxberg, Joseph D., M.D. *Bypass: A Doctor's Recovery from Open Heart Surgery.* New York: Appleton-Century-Crofts, 1981.

Wilber, Ken. *Eye to Eye.* New York: Anchor Books, 1983.

INDEX

A

Abandonment, fear of, 66, 219, 234-235, 244, 249, 276

Adapting, 44

Advocacy, 17-23, 123-125, 185-186, 240. _See also_ Communica tion; Patient advo- cate

American Association of Cardiovascular and Pulmonary Rehabili- tation, 99

American Heart Association, 99, 223

Aneurysm, 313 _defined_

Angelou, Maya, On The Pulse of Morning, 180

Anger, 44, 158-160, 202. _See also_ Feelings; Grief; Healing; Pain
  acknowledging, 159-162
  and blame, 159
  checklist, 75
  in communication, 74-75
  and disintegration, 159
  forgiving, 173-175
  as mask for fear, 70-71
  misdirected, 73
  the ogre, 70-75
  and release, 158, 201
  usefulness of, 73

Angina, 313 _defined_

Angiogram, 10, 27, 313-314 _defined_

Angioplasty, xvii, 10

Antiarrhyrhmics, 317 _defined_

Anticoagulants, 317 _defined_

Antihypertensives, 317 _defined_

Anxiety, 65, _See also_ Fear; Feelings; Sleep
  and change, 47-48
  chronic, 68
  and denial, xxiii
  easing of, 13, 69-70
  the great paralyzer, 63-64
  numbness, 64, 198
  symptoms of, 11, 201
  and travel, 48-50
  and trembling, 11, 65
  and the unknown, 14

Aorta, 314 _defined_

Appetite, 11, 35
  and your role, 52-53

Appreciation
  lack of, 35

Arguing, 34-35

Arrhythmia, 314 _defined_

Arteries, 314 _defined_
  See also Coronary arteries

Arterioschlerosis, 314 _defined_

Atherosclerosis, 314 _defined_

B

Balloon angioplasty, 314 _defined_

Beginning, a new, 150

of intimacy, 130
and pain, 155-156
physical comfort, 231-234
of poverty, 67
and responsibility, 127-
129
and sex, 210, 224-234
and seeking information,
67
survival, 129-130
unresolved, xxi
Feelings, 58, 82-85. *See also*
Anger; Anxiety;
Cardiackids;
Change; Crisis;
Dependency; Depres-
sion; Fear; Forgive
ness; Grief; Healing;
Helplessness; Imag-
ery; Mourning;
Nightmares; Opti-
mism; Pain;
Positive; Responsibil-
ity; Roles;
Sadness; Scars; Self-
help tools; Spiritual-
ity; Story; Stress;
Support; Tension;
Uncertainty; Visual
ization; Vulnerability;
Wounds
acknowledging, 158-162
arguing, 34-35
assessment diary, 83
compassion, 123-125
confusion, 4, 24
control, 4, 34, 52, 63, 106,
131-132, 147
covering up, 181
denial of, 60
despair, 142

disproportion of 14
distance, 60
embarrassment, 44
as energy drain, 61
of failure, 142
guidance, 5
guilt, 33, 63
and hospital, 15
and life-style changes, 44
mistaken for stress, 136
and pain, 155-156
of patient, 61-62
points to remember, 82
releasing, 158-162, 181
resentment, 134-135, 140
sadness, 76-80
seeking support, 85, 265-
266
steps to change, 82-83
taking stock, 69-70
trivializing, 154
wounds, 147-180
Finances. *See also* Role;
Work
accepting support, 87
and new reality, 149, 195
changing status of, 39-43,
55
and discussion, 40-43
and family business, 57
responsibility, 54-55
Food. *See also* Control; Diet;
Sodium
and change, 54
cheating, 34-35
efforts to please, 35
issues, 35-36
as love, 33
nutritionist, 22
Forgiveness, 173-175, 232,
234, 238

Heartmates® is an ongoing therapeutic program designed to serve the cardiac spouse and family during and after a cardiac crisis. To be included on our mailing list, please print your name and address below and mail to:

Heartmates, Inc.
P.O. Box 16202
Minneapolis, MN 55416

Or write your questions and concerns to us via e-mail at:
heartmates@aol.com
or the WorldWideWeb: http://www.heartmates.com/

Your age now: _____ Your spouse's age: _____
Date of onset of heart disease: _____
What has changed most in *your* life since the onset of your mate's heart disease? _____

_____

What concerns you most right now? _____

_____

_____.

A Videoseries, *Portrait of a Heartmate*; each of five-20 minute programs focuses on a different topic. Titles are: *"After A Heart Attack," "Understanding Cardiac Care," "The Road To Recovery," "Family Concerns," and "Renewing The Relationship."* This series is available for personal use and costs US $59.95, including shipping and handling.

A new interactive and user-friendly resource; *The Heartmates® Meditation Journal: A Daily Companion for Partners of Heart Patients.* This yearlong aid focuses on the changes in the heartmate's life when a partner has heart disease. A beautiful edition, *The Heartmates Meditation Journal* makes a wonderful gift and will fit in purse or briefcase...a support companion you will want to use daily. US $15.00, including shipping and handling.

Heartmates® Inc. will accept personal checks or money orders; NO credit cards are available ...

❑ Portrait of a Heartmate Videoseries $59.95
❑ The Heartmates® Meditation Journal: A Daily Companion $15.00

NAME _____

ADDRESS _____

CITY _____ STATE _____

ZIP CODE _____ PHONE (____) _____

call (800) 9HM-3331 for more information or your questions

Heartmates® is an ongoing therapeutic program designed to serve the cardiac spouse and family during and after a cardiac crisis. To be included on our mailing list, please print your name and address below and mail to:

Heartmates, Inc.
P.O. Box 16202
Minneapolis, MN 55416

Or write your questions and concerns to us via e-mail at:
heartmates@aol.com
or the WorldWideWeb: http://www.heartmates.com/

Your age now: _____ Your spouse's age: _____
Date of onset of heart disease: _____
What has changed most in *your* life since the onset of your mate's heart disease? _____
_____

What concerns you most right now? _____
_____
_____
_____.

A Videoseries, *Portrait of a Heartmate*; each of five-20 minute programs focuses on a different topic. Titles are: *"After A Heart Attack," "Understanding Cardiac Care," "The Road To Recovery," "Family Concerns," and "Renewing The Relationship."* This series is available for personal use and costs US $59.95, including shipping and handling.

A new interactive and user-friendly resource; *The Heartmates® Meditation Journal: A Daily Companion for Partners of Heart Patients.* This yearlong aid focuses on the changes in the heartmate's life when a partner has heart disease. A beautiful edition, *The Heartmates Meditation Journal* makes a wonderful gift and will fit in purse or briefcase...a support companion you will want to use daily. US $15.00, including shipping and handling.

Heartmates® Inc. will accept personal checks or money orders; NO credit cards are available ...

❏ Portrait of a Heartmate Videoseries $59.95
❏ The Heartmates® Meditation Journal: A Daily Companion $15.00

NAME _____
ADDRESS _____
CITY _____ STATE _____
ZIP CODE _____ PHONE (____) _____

call (800) 9HM-3331 for more information or your questions